Volume 4

PLANS AND PROVISIONS FOR THE MENTALLY HANDICAPPED

PLANS AND PROVISIONS FOR THE MENTALLY HANDICAPPED

MARGARET BONE, BERNIE SPAIN AND F. M. MARTIN

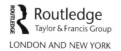

LONDON AND NEW YORK

First published in 1972 by George Allen & Unwin Ltd

This edition first published in 2022
by Routledge
2 Park Square, Milton Park, Abingdon, Oxon OX14 4RN

and by Routledge
605 Third Avenue, New York, NY 10158

Routledge is an imprint of the Taylor & Francis Group, an informa business

British Library Cataloguing in Publication Data
A catalogue record for this book is available from the British Library

ISBN: 978-1-03-203381-5 (Set)
ISBN: 978-1-00-321681-0 (Set) (ebk)
ISBN: 978-1-03-206000-2 (Volume 4) (hbk)
ISBN: 978-1-03-206008-8 (Volume 4) (pbk)
ISBN: 978-1-00-320021-5 (Volume 4) (ebk)

DOI: 10.4324/9781003200215

Publisher's Note
The publisher has gone to great lengths to ensure the quality of this reprint but points out that some imperfections in the original copies may be apparent.

This book is a re-issue originally published in 1972. The language used is reflective of its era and no offence is meant by the Publishers to any reader by this re-publication.

Disclaimer
The publisher has made every effort to trace copyright holders and would welcome correspondence from those they have been unable to trace.

PLANS AND PROVISIONS
FOR THE
MENTALLY HANDICAPPED

MARGARET BONE
BERNIE SPAIN
and
F. M. MARTIN

WITH A PREFACE BY
DR GUY WIGLEY
Deputy Medical Adviser,
Greater London Council

London
GEORGE ALLEN & UNWIN LTD
RUSKIN HOUSE   MUSEUM STREET

First published 1972

ISBN 0 04 362023 X

PRINTED IN GREAT BRITAIN
in 11 point Baskerville type
by Clarke, Doble & Brendon Ltd.
Plymouth

MEMBERS OF STEERING COMMITTEE

ACKNOWLEDGEMENTS

In the course of writing, we talked to many people who were helpful to us, but in particular we should like to thank Dr Albert Kushlick who gave us much encouragement and constructive criticism. We would also like to thank Professor J. Tizard and his research staff at the Institute of Education, Dr Brian Kirman, Elspeth Stephens, Dr George Brown, Dr Joyce Leeson, Dr Gordon Rose and Mrs Winifred Curzon. Needless to say none of these people can be held responsible for any of the opinions or interpretations of data expressed here.

We always received much help from the Department of Health and Social Security (then the Ministry of Health), who generously gave us access to unpublished records and helped us with difficulties in interpreting figures. We are also extremely grateful to the fifteen Regional Hospital Boards, to all the hospitals for the mentally handicapped which co-operated in the research, particularly those in the three Regions where we undertook the ward studies, and to the Medical Officers of Health and their staffs, in the nine Boroughs which formerly comprised Middlesex, who allowed us access to the records of former Middlesex patients whose records we wished to trace.

M.B.
B.S.
F.M.M.

PREFACE

BY DR GUY WIGLEY

Deputy Medical Adviser, Greater London Council

———

This study, sponsored by the National Association for Mental Health, the National Society for Mentally Handicapped Children and the Spastics Society, arose from discussions following the publication of *A Hospital Plan for England and Wales*.

The policy paragraph in that document dealing with the number of hospital beds required for the mentally handicapped is notably weak; after weighing factors which might lead to the need for more beds against those tending to require less, the concluding sentence reads: 'Provisionally it has been assumed that eventually the factors mentioned above will more or less offset one another, but plans may need radical alteration in one direction or another as time time goes on.' Not, one thinks, a sound statement on which plans can, with confidence, be based. Statistical studies of bed requirements are clearly needed, and it is unrealistic to look at the need for hospital beds in isolation from community provision, since many of the mentally handicapped can be cared for in either situation. Energetic development of good-quality community services must reduce the need for hospital beds. It was therefore decided to study the services for the mentally handicapped in the round and in the expectation that the enquiry would go some way to provide a firmer foundation for the planning of services.

The study was guided by a steering committee, composed of representatives of the three societies and others with a special knowledge of mentally handicapped, of which I was chairman. The field work was undertaken by two research officers, Mrs Margaret Bone, B.Sc. (Soc.), and Miss Bernie Spain, M.A., Dip. Psych. F. M. Martin, Ph.D., at that time Reader in Social Medicine at the University of Edinburgh, acted as research consultant.

This work was originally designed to take two years, but access to full record material made available by the Middle-

sex County Health Department justified detailed analysis of
a kind which is new in this country. In the end the study took
nearly three years to complete and has since then had to be
put into book form.

This is primarily a statistical study and does not contain
case studies either of individual patients or of individual hospitals. Its purpose is not to expose but rather to make a con-
tribution to that knowledge on which alone sound plans can
be based. Those concerned with it have, however, been made
very aware of the problems with which hospital staff are
valiantly struggling, including widespread lack of facilities for
themselves and their patients. They have also become con-
vinced of the need for very close working between the hospitals
and the Local Authorities whose areas they serve, for long-
term planning no less than on a day-to-day basis.

Basically this work comprises four statistical studies : a census
of patients in all hospitals for the mentally handicapped in
England and Wales; a sample enquiry to ascertain the characteristics of hospital patients in some detail, the degree of mental
and physical handicap, their employment and training (the
Ward Study); a study of the subsequent experience of patients
first admitted to hospitals in one Hospital Region in 1949,
1959 and 1963, which demonstrates how the proportionate use
of hospitals by successive intakes has dramatically declined,
although the number of admissions has greatly increased; and
lastly, a cohort study of the subsequent experience of all first
referrals to the Middlesex Health Department for mental
handicap, which shows how a notable increase in the provision
of community training paralleled not only a decline in hospital
care but also a fall in the waiting-list.

The authors have not limited themselves to the compilation
of statistics but have also commented on various matters concerning the organization of the National Health Service, both
now and in the future. They discuss the treatment and training
of patients, the role and training of nurses, and the future of
Local Authority care.

While fully realizing the importance of strengthening community services Mrs Bone and Miss Spain recognize the importance of the hospital and of the burdens it must bear in
caring for cases of increasingly severe handicap – often multiple
– for many years to come. Their constructive conclusions are

particularly welcome at a time when ill-informed and hasty criticism has had a demoralizing effect on staff.

In their final chapter the authors comment on the 'incidental evidence' that in the main the authorities responsible for local health and hospital regional administrative statistics keep their records in such a way that only information demanded of them by the Department of Health is readily available – for the keeping of records for service planning is expensive. When these authorities publish figures relating to services in their own area, it is usually those which are returned to the Department that are printed. In other words the returns required by the Department to a large extent determine what information is available to local decision-makers. Apart from the planning of services, the information sought by a central department can also act as a useful guide at local level as to the quality of services, and good questions can trigger off productive trains of thought. It is clear that the central Government can, by calling for the right kind of statistical information, influence and stimulate the thinking of Regional Hospital Boards and Local Health Authorities. If the Department of Health and Social Security, which has contributed financially to this study, takes the hint, it will be interesting to see what questions they ask of local units in the future.

CONTENTS

TABLES

DIAGRAMS

I

MENTAL HANDICAP AS A
HOSPITAL AND COMMUNITY PROBLEM

This study arose from a concern with the adequacy of services
for the mentally handicapped. At the time we commenced the
project a good deal of research and investigation was in progress into various aspects of hospital and community services
for the mentally ill. The facilities provided for the mentally
handicapped, however, have always attracted less, and certainly much less well-publicized research. There has been an
increasing acceptance, at any rate among the educated public,
of the view that mental illness is a hazard from which no one
could assume himself to be wholly immune. But mental handicap can very rarely be considered in any ordinary sense a
condition which one acquires. There is a small risk that healthy
adults will produce mentally handicapped children, but this
is a chance that seems to concern most people – if indeed it
does at all – only during those relatively brief periods of anxiety
that precede childbirth. In addition, mental handicap does
not yield to dramatic cures, is usually depressing to contem-
plate and, unlike mental illness, is never the subject of fascinat-
ing psychological or literary speculation. Consequently the level
of public interest in mental handicap appears in general to be
relatively low.

More recently, with the publication of the Ely Report
(1969), there has been more public discussion of the problems
of the mentally handicapped, and more regard given to the
fact that these citizens have not in the past received the attention and resources which are needed if they and their families
are to achieve the standards of comfort and freedom which are
their right. Over the last year or two more consideration has
been given to these issues, and in particular to the situation
of the mentally handicapped who cannot live in their own
homes. However, because of the low level of interest in them

over past years, little statistical material has been available until recently about mentally handicapped patients or their needs.

Over 60,000 mentally handicapped patients are housed at present in hospitals in England and Wales. At the national level there is little information about the characteristics of these patients and only speculation about the way in which the resident population may change in the future. During a period when the planning of future hospital requirements has been much discussed, this seems to be a serious gap in knowledge. Not only the absolute number, but the type of patient involved greatly affects the kind of accommodation, staffing and facilities required. Patients of very low intelligence with physical handicaps, who may spend the rest of their lives in hospital, have very different requirements from high-grade patients with behaviour problems who need rehabilitation, and different again from medium-grade patients, who may or may not be able to return to the community, but who are mostly trainable. Recently there have been several publications from the Wessex Regional Hospital Board study, which was partly financed by the Department of Health. These give details of inpatient characteristics which should be generalizable to the country as a whole. Pauline Morris's report *Put Away* also gives some details of inpatient characteristics in the sample of hospitals she studied. However, there is still quite inadequate knowledge of patient turnover or of the factors which influence the decision to admit or discharge patients.

In January 1962 a Hospital Plan for England and Wales was published (Ministry of Health, 1962). This collected together the separate plans for hospital development produced by the fifteen Regional Hospital Boards in the country for a period of fifteen years (1960–75) and was complemented by a similar plan for the development of community services by the (then) 146 Local Health Authorities. Commenting on the provision of beds for the mentally handicapped, the authors of the Hospital Plan pointed out that the bed provision which should be made by 1975 was difficult to estimate. They suggested various factors which might influence need in conflicting ways and concluded by making the tentative assumption that these would offset one another, so that no change in the level of provision need be anticipated. Such assumptions are hardly an adequate basis for designing an effective hospital service

(Rehin and Martin, 1963). A better basis can only be constructed by the provision of more information about the mentally handicapped and their needs.

The present study arose from concern about these deficiencies in the Hospital Plan and had two principal aims in view : firstly to examine the characteristics of the resident hospital population and secondly to enquire into recent changes in the numbers, characteristics and outcome of patients admitted to hospital, and what changes, if any, in community services have influenced these. The general intention of this approach is to provide information which can be used as a basis on which to assess the effectiveness of services and as a means of predicting future needs.

Because of the primarily quantitative nature of the material used in this report, there will be little reference to the practical consequences of inadequate services for individual people. Perhaps therefore it should be emphasized at the outset that the adequacy or otherwise of residential accommodation has far-reaching effects upon the families of many defective patients as well as upon the patients themselves. During the course of this study we encountered much distress resulting from the failure of services to provide for particular needs : marriages which had apparently broken down because the patient's presence at home imposed too great a strain on the relationship; mothers who, having made the difficult decision to place the subnormal child in hospital in the interests of other children in the family, found that there was no hope of the patient being admitted for several years; there were other cases where the child was eventually admitted, only to be taken from the hospital by his parents shortly afterwards because they considered that the hospital environment produced a deterioration in the child's condition. We quote these examples not because they are typical – we do not know that they are – but because they illustrate the kind of situation and the problems which made the study necessary.

RECENT ATTITUDES TO SUBNORMALITY SERVICES

Although public interest in the problem of the mentally handicapped has only recently been aroused, over the past decade or so more attention has been paid to this subject by research workers and practitioners, not only in this country, but also in other parts of Europe and in the U.S.A. It seems important to discuss briefly some of the issues which have been raised because the results of the present study have some bearing on them.

In the post-war period the idea has developed that mentally handicapped patients might be cared for better and achieve a greater degree of social and economic independence if they lived in the community rather than in hospital. This view arose in Britain as a belated reaction to the attitudes enshrined in the Mental Deficiency Act of 1913, passed at least in part to enable high-grade defectives to be placed in custodial care, for fear lest their freedom to propagate should contribute to national degeneracy (Hilliard and Kirman, 1965). The newer approach is based primarily on the results of more sophisticated genetic research, but in addition observations of the effects of environment on intelligence and the success of training programmes in improving the social competence of defectives have also led to more optimistic attitudes.

The view that the mentally handicapped should remain in the community has usually related to high- and medium-grade patients. However, the Royal Commission, reporting in 1957, recommended that hospitals should provide care for 'helpless patients in the severely subnormal group who need continual nursing *if* proper care cannot be provided at home' together with 'in-patient training . . . for severely subnormal and psychopathic patients *if* such training requires individual psychiatric supervision' (our italics). In other words, the Royal Commission considered that, even for the most handicapped and disturbed patients, hospital accommodation should be provided only when medical, psychiatric or full nursing care was necessary and could not be provided elsewhere. Even before the Mental Health Act of 1959 or the Royal Commission Report two years before, there had been a gradual expansion of community services for the mentally handicapped, and during the 1960s Local Authority services continued to develop at an accelerated rate. In particular there has been a growth in residential accommodation provided by Local Authorities, especially since 1960 (Ministry of Health, Annual Reports 1960-9), as an alternative to hospital care, and an increase in the number of special care units which provide day care for the very handicapped and low-grade patients. Although these services originally expanded as a result of the positive belief that community care was preferable to hospital care, the trend may to some extent have been strengthened by purely practical considerations, such as the size of the waiting-list and the sheer inability of hospitals to cope with the increased demand which a growing population alone placed upon them. By 1959, however, and as with the mentally ill, the assumption had clearly been made that keeping patients within the community was the right and proper objective.

Although there can be no doubt that the intention is humanitarian, it is of dubious value to implement a policy of retaining the mentally handicapped in the community without at the same time examining the effect of this on the patients and, equally important, on his family. In the field of chronic mental illness, for example, Brown and his colleagues (1966) have shown that a policy of retaining schizophrenic patients in the community can lead to an increase in problems for their families even where community services are provided. Only careful study can reveal what kind and what level of services are required to allow patients to live outside hospital without placing undue strain on their families. This is not to say that changes should never be made in services without elaborate prior experiment, but that where such experimentation is not practicable, then, at the very least, the consequences which follow from administrative decisions should be observed, monitored and analysed.

A further issue concerns the mixing of patients of different grades. It was recommended to the Royal Commission (Minutes of Evidence, 1954) that high-grade and low-grade patients should be treated differently and housed separately, particularly if the former are within the normal I.Q. range. Subsequent research (Stein and Susser, 1960; Leeson 1963) has developed this argument, and it was reiterated in the Hospital Plan. It is not clear, however, to what extent this policy has been put into effect, and indeed there may actually have been an increase in the number of patients of normal I.Q. admitted to subnormality hospitals over recent years (Craft and Miles, 1967).

Another controversy concerns the best way in which to organize residential care for long-stay patients who obviously require a different environment from the acutely ill. As far as is possible long-stay establishments should provide patients with home-like surroundings. This is particularly true for the mentally handicapped who in the main are not 'sick' at all, but merely slow learners or backward. This viewpoint has been developed in the work of Tizard (1964) and Kushlick (1967), who have pioneered the idea that subnormal children who require residential care are best placed in small 'family units' similar to those considered most suitable for normal children unable to live at home. As a result, the advantages are being explored of a different approach to the organization of children's wards (Stephens, 1972) and of the development of small homes for children within the community, as an alternative to hospital admission (Kushlick, 1967). A somewhat conflicting viewpoint is expressed by McKeown in his concept of the district general hospital (Leck, Gordon and McKeown, 1967), in which it is envisaged that the mentally subnormal and other long-stay patients will be housed under the same roof, if they require hospital care, as acutely ill patients requiring surgical or medical treatment. To apply either method of care more widely and to determine which would be most appropriate in different Regions, it would be useful to have much greater knowledge than is presently available on the inpatient population, especially for children, and of the effect on the demand for residential care of providing more effective community services.

Interest in the conditions under which subnormal inpatients live has given rise to a further controversy about hospital size. Reformers have generally argued that large hospitals, however well-intentioned their administration, inevitably produce a degree of standardization in the treatment of patients, and in the organization of wards and staff which makes it difficult for patients to achieve maximum freedom and independence (Pilkington, 1963; Tizard, 1964; Mathews, 1969). On the other hand, it is claimed that only a large hospital can provide the variety of services which make comprehensive care of patients possible (Shapiro, 1963, 1969; McCoull, 1965. While the present study is not specifically concerned with resolving this problem, it is obviously important, in moving towards a solution, to know among other things what kind of services and training are likely to be required by hospital inpatients and whether these are such that large units are essential.

SOME QUESTIONS TO BE ANSWERED

The officially published statistics of admissions to and discharges from hospitals for the mentally retarded have till recently, at least been less illuminating than they might have been. They were examined at the beginning of the present enquiry, and the main findings of that examination are set out in the following chapter. On the whole we found that the published statistics raised more questions than they resolved, and these unanswered questions formed the starting-point of our own researches, so it may be helpful to set out briefly what were the questions which seemed to us to be of primary concern.

In the first place we thought it would be useful to gain some information on inpatient characteristics which would supplement the data published by the Department of Health's Annual Reports and in the Department's inpatient census (Brooke, 1963). We decided to do this by looking at a sample survey of patients in three hospital Regions. Secondly, since there was no published information on hospital facilities, training, teaching etc., we attempted a national survey of subnormality hospitals to gain some idea of what facilities are provided in relation to the type of patient they house. We also used this opportunity to test whether our sample survey appeared to represent the national inpatient population, by comparing them on simple demographic factors, such as age and sex.

However, we also thought it necessary to consider what changes had occurred in the demand for and the use of hospital care, since in this respect official statistics are particularly deficient. What actually happened after 1959 when the Mental Health Act came into force? Did admissions really show a sharp increase, as Department of Health figures suggest (see Diagram 2.3) and, if so, what type of patient accounted for the increase? Even for the earlier years, when fuller details were published, it is still not clear which kind of patient was being discharged, since the statistical tables showing length of stay for discharged patients gave no analyses by age and grade.

In order to find out what has happened to patients admitted

to hospital during a particular period of time and how this differs from the experience of patients admitted during another period, that is to discover what trends are affecting and will affect the demands made on hospitals, a cohort analysis of admissions is necessary.[1] Consequently we undertook an analysis of patients admitted to one hospital Region, in the years 1949, 1959 and 1963, to discover their characteristics in relation to the changing patterns of discharge, to discuss how patterns of hospitalization had changed and to detect whether any of these could be attributed to changes in policy, and in particular to the 1959 Mental Health Act.

A further problem we sought to answer was why, if the published statistics are correct, the total number of admissions to hospital increased at a time when community services were also apparently increasing (see Diagrams 2.1 and 2.3). It might be assumed that improved community provision would affect the demand for hospital care, but is this so and, if it is, what kind of services are important and for what types of patient? In order to throw more light on this issue we undertook a cohort study of referrals to one Local Authority, Middlesex, hoping to see how demand for hospital care had changed over time, and to see if this could be related at all to improved community services. As far as we are aware, no similar studies (i.e. cohort studies) of subnormal referrals or admissions have been undertaken in this country.

The following chapters contain the results of our studies, and questions arising, whose answers fall outside the scope of the present study and require further research, are discussed in the conclusion.

[1] The term 'cohort analysis' is widely used in actuarial and demographic studies. A cohort is a series of persons defined by a common experience in a particular period of time – for example, everyone born in 1930, everyone married in 1960, everyone admitted to hospital in 1965. A cohort analysis examines statistically the subsequent experiences of the members of different cohorts; for example one might calculate the number of marriages terminated by divorce five, ten and fifteen years after marriage, comparing the experience of those whose marriages were celebrated in 1930, 1940 and 1950.

2

THE OFFICIAL STATISTICS OF MENTAL HANDICAP: THEIR USES AND LIMITATIONS

HISTORICAL BACKGROUND

In England and Wales hospital services for the mentally handicapped are provided by the Regional Hospital Boards, while Local Government Departments provide services for patients in the community. Public hospitals for psychiatric patients were developed during the latter half of the nineteenth century when many of the existing institutions were built. In 1948 they were incorporated together with many of the voluntary hospitals into the National Health Service (N.H.S.), when they became the direct responsibility of the fourteen, now fifteen, Regional Hospital Boards of England and Wales.

Until 1952, admission to hospital involved almost without exception a formal legal procedure, but in that year informal short-term admission for periods of up to eight weeks was given official encouragement. The Royal Commission on the Law relating to Mental Illness and Mental Deficiency was appointed soon after; it reported in 1957 and recommended that in future hospital care for mentally ill and mentally handicapped patients should always be provided without formality, except where detention was unavoidable This proposal was implemented in 1958 and in the following year the Mental Health Act (1959) made the use of informal admission procedures legally explicit. By 1968, 90 per cent (9,327 out of 10,286) of mentally handicapped patients were admitted without formality whilst 93 year cent (60,783 out of 64,783) of patients in hospital were resident without legal compulsion.

The Mental Deficiency Act of 1927 required Local Authorities, who at that time administered hospitals, to provide training or occupation for resident patients. At the present time there is no specific obligation upon hospitals to provide training although the Royal Commission stressed that hospitals should give training devised to make the patient better equipped to live in the community. Subsequently the Department of Health and Social Security has sought to encourage industrial therapy and other forms of education in training.

Provision for the mentally handicapped in the community rests with the Local Authority Health and Social Service Departments. This dates from the Mental Deficiency Act of 1913 which stipulated that Local Authorities should ascertain which persons in their area were mentally defective and 'subject to be dealt with', and provide supervision for those who did not require admission to institutions or guardianship. The Mental Deficiency Act of 1927 added to this the duty of providing suitable training or occupation for patients who were under supervision unless there were adequate reasons for not doing so. In 1948 the National Health Service Act enabled Local Authorities to provide community care for defectives who were not under statutory supervision.

The Royal Commission of 1954–7 recommended a general shift of emphasis from hospital to community care, and proposed that it should be a duty for Local Authorities to provide training for all subnormal patients in their area. These recommendations were given force by the 1959 Mental Health Act and further promoted by the plan for community care published in 1963 (Ministry of Health, 1963 a). The number of patients undergoing training in the community has, in fact, shown a steady increase at least since 1952 (when the figures were first published), and the main effect of the later legislation was to extend training facilities for patients over the age of 16 (who form the majority of patients in the community). This has shown a particularly steep rise since 1961 (Diagram 2.1). By the end of 1968, however, nearly one-third of those aged 16 and over in the care of Local Authorities were receiving training compared with about 70 per cent of patients aged less than 16 years (D.H.S.S. Annual Report, 1968). However, an unknown percentage of adult patients in the community may be in paid employment or too old to be suitable for training.[1]

[1] The responsibility for training mentally handicapped children has now been transferred from the Department of Health to the Department of Education and Science.

In addition to training, the 1959 Act enabled Local Authorities to provide residential accommodation for patients in the community, and by the end of 1968 about 5 per cent of patients outside hospital were resident at the Local Authorities' expense in nursing-homes or private households.

Despite the increased efforts of Local Authorities to provide services for patients living at home, there seems to have been very little change in the percentage of subnormals resident in the community. In 1968 some 60 per cent (99,820 out of 164,603) of all officially recognized subnormals were resident in the community compared with approximately 62 per cent in 1955 (source – Ministry of Health Annual Reports, 1955 and D.H.S.S. Annual Report, 1968). This suggests either that increased community provision up to 1968 had produced no effect on admissions to hospital, or that other factors were

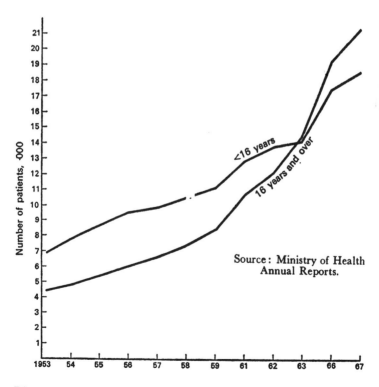

Diagram 2.1   Number of patients receiving training in the community in England and Wales, between 1953 and 1967

operating to offset the effect. However, the comparison may not be valid, because, as we shall show later, hospital residents before and after 1960 are differently defined.

CLASSIFICATION OF THE MENTALLY HANDICAPPED

Before the Mental Health Act of 1959, three grades of mental handicap were distinguished. These were legally defined mainly according to criteria of social competence, but were commonly understood to represent three I.Q. groups (Tizard, 1965). The term 'idiot' referred to those whose I.Q. fell roughly below 20 or 25 points and 'imbecile' to those whose I.Q. lay approximately between 25 and 50 points. Those with I.Q.s between 50 and 70 were termed 'feeble-minded' although people within this I.Q. range were not usually classified as feeble-minded unless other circumstances besides low intelligence brought them to notice.

The 1959 Act abolished these terms on the recommendation of the Royal Commission and substituted two grades for the former three: 'subnormality' and 'severe subnormality' (revised recently to 'mentally handicapped' and 'severely mentally handicapped').[2] Although these terms, unlike the earlier ones, include a specific reference to subnormality of intelligence, there are several disadvantages in their use. First, confusion arises because all patients are called by the general term of 'the mentally subnormal', or nowadays 'the mentally handicapped', while at the same time the terms 'subnormal' or 'mentally handicapped' refers only to those at the higher end of the I.Q. scale.

Secondly, there is as yet no consensus on the range of intelligence covered by each grade. Although in general 'mentally handicapped' or 'subnormal' is considered to be equivalent to the former term 'feeble-minded' and 'severely mentally handicapped' to the former imbecile and idiot grades, *in practice* there appears to be no agreement on the boundaries between the two groups. (Castell, *et al.*, 1963.)

The major distinction is still maintained between high-grade

---

[2] In addition, patients classified as 'psychopaths' (formerly termed 'moral defectives') may be admitted to subnormality hospitals, as well as to hospitals for the mentally ill, regardless of their level of intelligence.

patients, who may well be capable of leading an independent life, given the correct training, and lower-grade patients who are most unlikely ever to be able to do so. But as Clarke and Clarke have pointed out, because the Mental Health Act 'makes it much easier to detain compulsorily patients over the age of 25 if they are severely subnormal' . . . there is . . . 'an obvious temptation to use this category in the case of difficult patients, a temptation that is apparently not always resisted' (Clarke and Clarke, 1965). Consequently it cannot be assumed that all patients categorized as severely subnormal are in fact incapable of leading an independent life, since they might be so designated for legal convenience. This presumably accounts for the findings in a special study carried out for the British Psychological Society (Castell et al., 1963). Hospital psychologists were asked to test all patients on admission and compare test results with the designations given. The average I.Q. of the 'severely subnormal' or 'severely mentally handicapped' was 60·4, i.e. well into the high-grade or feeble-minded range. In addition it is evident that quite a number of patients designated as 'subnormal' or 'mentally handicapped' have I.Q.s within the normal limits, since the mean I.Q. of subnormal patients in the study was 71. Many such patients therefore do not suffer from subnormality of intelligence in the generally accepted sense.

More importantly, there are now only two categories in which to consider patients rather than the former three. The nomenclature of the 1959 Act does not allow for the distinction between those patients so severely affected as to be totally dependent, or as the 1913 Act states 'unable to guard themselves against common physical dangers', and those who, although of low intelligence, are amenable to training at least to the extent of caring for their own basic needs, such as washing and dressing etc. When considering the needs of patients in residential care, the kind of behaviour that can be expected of them and the kind of staff required to care for them, this is a distinction which must be made.

In the present report therefore we have preferred to use a three-fold classification into high, medium and low (corresponding to the old concepts of feeble-minded, imbecile and idiot) and we add a fourth category, normal in intelligence, wherever the data available made this possible. In Chapter 4, however, we have kept to the 1913 terminology, and a brief explanation of why this was done is given at the beginning of that chapter. Because so many different classifications are used in different studies it might be useful to note here the various terms used in this and other studies and their rough equivalents in intelligence quotient, see Table 2.1.

TABLE 2.1

EQUIVALENT TERMS USED IN MENTAL DEFICIENCY
(AFTER KIRMAN, 1968, *British Medical Journal*)

General terms	Categories	IQ equivalent
	High grade	
	Subnormal	
	Feeble-minded	
	Mentally Handicapped	50–70
	Moron	
	Debile	
Mentally handicapped	Mildly retarded	
Mentally retarded	Educationally subnormal	
Mentally defective		
Mentally subnormal	Medium grade	
	Retarded	25–49
	Imbecile	
Severely	Trainable	
subnormal	Low grade	
Severely	Severely retarded	
mentally	Idiot	0–24
handicapped	Untrainable	

STATISTICAL TRENDS

Between 1949, when the National Health Service Act came into force, and 1960, two official sources of information on the hospital population were available: the Supplements on Mental Health to the Registrar General's Annual Reviews and the Annual Reports of the Chief Medical Officer, Ministry of Health (now the Department of Health and Social Security). The former gave analyses of admissions, discharges and deaths, while the Annual Reports showed the numbers resident in hospital. From 1961 onwards, following a recommendation of the Royal Commission, only the Department of Health has published inpatient statistics. These have been collected on a different basis from the previous period and, until 1969, were analysed in much less detail than those of the Registrar General. Except for the 1963 'Census of Patients in Psychiatric Beds' (Brooke, 1967), only very brief data were available between 1961 and 1969. More recently the situation has improved with the publication of the Department's Statistical Report Series and the Digest of Health Statistics, 1969. All these publications derive their material from the same basic sources – the 1963 Census, or the Mental Health Inquiry forms, completed for each patient on admission or discharge. However different statistical reports quote figures rather differently, and it is very difficult to piece together what has actually occurred over the course of time; whether any changes which appear when figures are compared between one year and the next represent actual changes in the hospital population or merely changes in the criteria for including material in the tables. In particular a major revision occurred in the definition of an inpatient in 1959, and consequently comparison of figures before and after 1960 is difficult to make. It is simplest therefore to consider the two periods separately.

CHANGES IN THE RESIDENT HOSPITAL POPULATION

1949–60

Both the General Register Office data and the Annual Report of the Chief Medical Officer give very similar totals for the number of patients resident in hospital over this time period. In 1949 approximately 54,000 inpatients were recorded and in the following decade this rose by 10 per cent to approximately 59,000. In 1956 hospitals were instructed to release patients who had been on licence in the community for more than eighteen months. Patients on licence had formerly been included as residents, and there was consequently a slight decline in the recorded hospital population for that year. Apart from this anomaly there was a steady rise in the numbers resident each year over this time period. No new large units for the mentally handicapped were built between 1949 and 1959 (although extensions to existing units were made), and it seems likely that most of the additional places were pro-

B

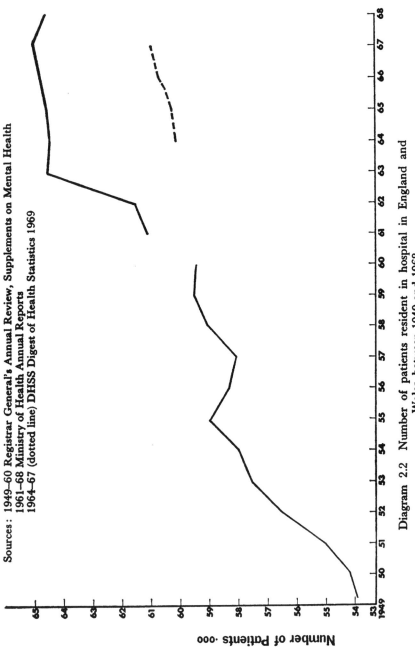

Diagram 2.2   Number of patients resident in hospital in England and Wales, between 1949 and 1968

Sources: 1949–60 Registrar General's Annual Review, Supplements on Mental Health
1961–68 Ministry of Health Annual Reports
1964–67 (dotted line) DHSS Digest of Health Statistics 1969

Number of Patients ·000

vided by increasing the nursing staff and putting more patients into existing accommodation. Many hospitals had of course been run down during the war years owing to staff shortages. Also a few additional hospitals were included in the later years as more units, still private in 1949, came under N.H.S. administration.

1961-8

Following the 1959 Mental Health Act, the Department of Health altered the criteria for counting a patient as resident in hospital. Previously only patients resident in establishments legally designated to receive the 'mentally deficient' were included, but the first census of psychiatric patients, carried out in April 1961, covered all patients with the diagnosis of 'subnormality' in N.H.S. beds, 'under the care of a psychiatrist', whatever the type of institution. The 1961 Census figures report an increase of approximately 2,000 over those shown in the 1959 Annual Report, although the annual increase up to that time had only been in the order of 500 a year. The December 1961 and 1962 figures quote similar totals, but a further large increase is reported for the 1963 Census, this time of over 3,000 to a total of 64,622.

It is probable that this apparent increase in residents was due largely to the change in the definition of a patient to be included in the tables. Up to 1961 patients in mental illness hospitals appeared in the statistics as 'mentally ill', regardless of diagnosis, but the 1963 Census revealed that some 6,000 patients with mental subnormality were present in hospitals for the mentally ill, and most, if not all, of these would not have been counted as mentally handicapped previously. According to figures in subsequent Annual Reports, based on updated Census figures, the number of patients resident has remained at approximately 64·6 thousand up to 1968, the last year for which figures for England and Wales were published together. (The figure from the 1969 Annual Report refers to English hospitals only, because from this year the health and welfare services in Wales became the responsibility of the Secretary of State for Wales.) The Digest of Health Statistics (1969) gives figures for the number of residents between 1964 and 1967, within various types of institutions, but appears to exclude those living in hospitals for the mentally ill. The Digest figures are in the order of 60·5 thousand, i.e. about 4,000 fewer than the figure quoted in the Annual Reports for the same period. One must conclude therefore that the number of mentally handicapped patients in hospital has probably changed very little since the 1959 Mental Health Act was passed, and that any apparent difference is probably due mainly to the inclusion in some tables of patients resident in mental illness hospitals.

There certainly does not seem to be any evidence of a decrease in the number of mentally handicapped living in hospital. Possibly there has been some increase, but it is difficult to determine this because of the different definitions used over time. It is not possible to be more definite than this because of the conflicting information present in different sets of statistics, and the fact that little if any comment accompanies the tables to help account for the discrepancies.[3]

COMPOSITION OF THE INPATIENT POPULATION

There have always been remarkably few details available in official sources about the characteristics of subnormal patients resident in hospital. The G.R.O. supplements analysed admissions and discharges by sex, age and grade, but classified inpatients only by sex (and in 1959 and 1960 by mental category, i.e. 'subnormal' and 'severely subnormal' equivalent to the new terms 'mentally handicapped' and 'severely mentally handicapped'). Apart from this no other information was collected or published except for the 1963 Census. This is very disappointing in its treatment of the mentally handicapped. Analyses of residents by sex and age are given and details of diagnosis are also provided, using the International Classification of Diseases. However this is not a very useful system, since the categories used confuse aetiological terms like phenylketonuria with classifications such as mongolism and schizophrenia and with the pre-1959 grades of defect, idiocy and imbecility. One cannot deduce from this system the capacities of patients, nor their degree of handicap, which might enable

---

[3] At the time of writing the Department of Health was responsible for all statistics on mental health, and it was not then possible for that Department to ascertain for us the precise coverage of figures published by the G.R.O. in former years.

one to predict the kind of inpatient services they are likely to require.

More useful information, however, is contained in the Report of the Royal Commission 1957, and details for limited areas can be found in various research reports – O'Connor and Tizard (1954), Leeson (1960) and Primrose (1966).

Most sources show very similar proportions of patients under 16 years (about 12 per cent). Comparing the 1957 and 1963 national data, no notable changes appear for patients aged under 55 years, although there were rather fewer patients in the age group 25–44 in 1963. The main trend which appears is in the proportion of older patients resident in hospital. There are twice as many patients aged 55 years and over in the later years than in 1954 (see Table 2.2).

TABLE 2.2

PERCENTAGE OF PATIENTS RESIDENT IN HOSPITAL,
BY AGE GROUP, IN VARIOUS STUDIES

Age groups		0–4	5–15	16–24	25–34	35–44	45–54	55+
Royal Commission	1954	0·7	11·3	20·8	24·3	19·4	16·1	9·4
Joyce Leeson	1959	0	6·3	23·3	19·2	19·5	16·9	12·7
Ministry census	1963	0·8	11·2	19·8	16·1	16·7	16·2	19·2
Primrose	1964	2·9	12·1	19·3	17·6	15·4	15·5	17·0

Note: The years in which the investigations were carried out are quoted, rather than the year of publication.

The proportion of patients in each of the three grades also shows important changes over the time period covered by the enquiries. O'Connor and Tizard's figures for London hospitals in 1952 and the 1954 national data given in the Royal Commission showed that about 6 per cent of the hospital population were low grade and 52 per cent were high grade at that time. Comparing this with figures given by Leeson (1959) and Primrose (1966), it appears that there has been an increase since the early 1950s in the proportion of low-grade patients in hospital, from 6 per cent to 17 per cent, and a corresponding decrease in the proportion of high-grade patients, from 52 to 30 per cent (see Table 2.3). If these changes reflect national trends it is important for the planning of services to know what factors have brought them about, and whether the same trends are likely to continue into the future.

TABLE 2.3

PERCENTAGE OF PATIENTS RESIDENT IN HOSPITAL,
BY GRADE, IN VARIOUS STUDIES

	O'Connor & Tizard 1952	Royal Commission 1954	Leeson 1959	Primrose 1964
Low grade	5·9	8	16·5	16·7
Medium grade	41·8	40	45·5	53·1
High grade	52·3	52	38·0	30·2

Note: The years in which the investigations were carried out are quoted, rather than the year of publication.

PATIENT MOVEMENT THROUGH HOSPITALS

The considerations which made difficult the comparison of patients resident before and after 1960 also apply to the figures for admissions, discharges and deaths. Diagram 2.3 shows that admissions apparently increased steadily but slowly until 1960 and then very steeply between 1960 and 1963, after which the rate of increase levelled off. (The peak in 1963 is due to the inclusion for this year alone of transfers between hospitals.) Part of the increase which occurred after 1960 is no doubt the result of the change in the definition of an inpatient which occurred after 1959 and has already been discussed. In the main, however, the rise seems to be due to the inclusion from that date of patients admitted for short-stay care (formerly called 5/52 admissions because the use of hospitals for short-stay care was first allowed in the Department Circular 5/52). These are patients admitted for a specified period, of up to two months but for no longer, to tide families over a crisis period or give them a short break from caring for the patient. This is obviously a very welcome service, since its use has mushroomed so rapidly over the last decade that by 1968 over half of all admissions (6,039 out of 10,904) were for short-stay care. The increase in long-term admissions has almost certainly risen much less sharply, and this pattern is apparent also in the cohort study of hospital admissions described in Chapter 5.

Discharges increased between 1956 (when a more liberal policy of discharge was introduced) and 1960, while the number of deaths remained more or less unchanged between

1949 and 1960. This must represent a lowered death rate since both admissions and the resident population were increasing during this period. Between 1960 and 1963 no separate figures for deaths and discharges were published, but figures are now available for the period 1964–6 (Department of Health, 1969).

These show that discharges have risen sharply, paralleling the rise in admissions, but much of this must be due to the

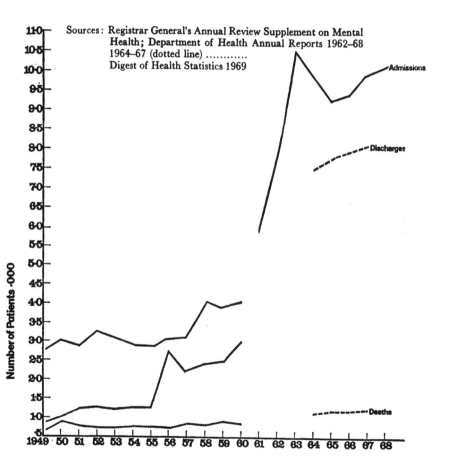

Diagram 2.3   Hospital admissions, discharges and deaths in England and Wales, between 1949 and 1967

Note: The figures for 1949–57 include statutory patients only; thereafter non-statutory patients are also included

discharge of patients admitted specifically for short-term care. The number of deaths appears to have risen also, but possibly this is due in part to the change in the definition of an inpatient; if the criteria for counting an inpatient as 'mentally handicapped' are broadened, then it follows that the number of patients dying who are said to be mentally handicapped would also increase.

ADMISSIONS, DEATHS, AND DISCHARGES BY AGE AND GRADE, 1949–60

Numbers of admissions for all age groups increased over the period except for patients aged 10–14 years. By far the largest increase in numbers is for patients aged 35 years and over – 12 per cent of all admissions in 1949 but 24 per cent in 1960.

Considering the grade of patient in relation to admissions and discharges, at least between 1953 and 1960 admissions of idiots and imbeciles exceeded the aggregate of discharges and deaths for these grades. For idiots, deaths accounted for most of the movement out of hospitals, but for imbeciles discharges exceeded deaths towards the end of the period. For the feeble-minded, discharges have greatly exceeded deaths at least since 1953.

An analysis of deaths by age and grade was first given by the G.R.O. in 1953, but was not subsequently provided for every year until 1958. In 1956 most of the imbeciles and feeble-minded patients who died were aged under 35 years, and most idiots under 15 years. In subsequent years most medium- and high-grade patients who died were 35 years or over and most idiots were 15 years or more, although the majority of these were under 20 years.

By contrast the age of discharged patients is shown to have fallen. Throughout the period most patients who were discharged were 25 years or older, but whereas in the earlier years about twice as many of the discharged patients were in the older group, by 1960 the older discharges were only about half as great again as the younger patients (1949, discharges aged 25 years and over = 604; under 25 years = 285; 1960, discharges aged 25 years and over = 1,886; under 25 years = 1,289). Most discharges under the age of 25 have been between 20 and 25.

Taken all together these figures support the evidence quoted earlier for an increase in the numbers and proportions of low-grade patients over the period and a decrease of high-grade patients. They do not throw light on the way in which the age structure of the hospital population might have changed.

RATES OF ADMISSION, 1949–60

Changes in the numbers of admissions, discharges and deaths give some indication of the changing demands on hospitals, but taken in isolation they do not show to what extent they reflect changes in the structure of the general population. An expansion of the population at risk will, other things being equal, give rise to an increased demand for services, although rates of admission remain stable. On the other hand changes in policy, incidence or prevalence may affect the number of patients admitted to hospital even in a stable population. It is therefore worthwhile to discover how far the increase in numbers of patients admitted to hospital is attributable to the increase in the general population.

Admission rates per million of home population between 1949 and 1960 showed considerable fluctuations, but that there was evidence for an overall increase in rates is fairly clear. Rates for males have always exceeded those for females by a fairly wide margin.

TABLE 2.4

HOSPITAL ADMISSION RATES IN ENGLAND AND WALES
PER MILLION AGE-RELATED POPULATION[1]

Age groups	1949–51	1958–60
0–4	82	90
5–9	144	164
10–14	180	124
15–19	249	295
20–24	83	132
25–34	48	76
35+	19	46

[1] Source: Registrar General's Annual Review.

Table 2.4 illustrates changes in rates for each age group. Rates for 1949–51 are compared with those for 1958–60. In this table 'accidental' or chance fluctuations are eliminated by the use of rates for three-year periods. The increased rate of admission occurred in most age groups, but not for patients aged between 10 and 15 years, for whom rates declined. Comparison with figures given for the United States by Sabagh and Windle (1959) for the years 1936–8 and 1953–5 is of interest, although the years covered differ. The overall pattern of age-specific rates is very similar. The American figures show a similar increase in rates for those aged under 10, and a slight fall for those aged 10–14. On the other hand they also show a decline for all ages over 15 years, unlike the figures for England and Wales.

TABLE 2.5

HOSPITAL ADMISSION RATES IN ENGLAND AND WALES, BY GRADE PER MILLION AGE-RELATED POPULATION[1]

Age groups	Low grade 1949–51	Low grade 1958–60	Medium grade 1949–51	Medium grade 1958–60	High grade 1949–51	High grade 1958–60
0–4	27	35	40	49	7	6
5–9	39	47	76	98	21	18
10–14	15	19	70	72	88	32
15–19	6	10	41	65	195	218
20–24	3	5	19	28	57	94
25–34	3	4	14	24	28	47
35+	1	3	7	20	10	23

[1] Source: Registrar General's Annual Review.

Examination of trends in age-specific rates, by grade, provides results which are of dubious value as a guide to the actual situation. In the earlier years the G.R.O. figures confounded grade with diagnosis and, in the later years, 'social reasons' for admission with grade. It has been assumed in the following analysis that, in the G.R.O. data, ungraded patients who were admitted for 'social reasons' were high-grade patients, but no assumptions can be made about the grading of patients classified by diagnosis, although it is likely that most of these were medium- or low-grade. Table 2.5 shows apparent trends in age-specific admission rates for the three grades. No comparable figures can be derived for the period 1964–6. The decline in admissions for patients aged 10–14 occurs only amongst the high-grades, but there was also a slight decline in rates of admission for the high-grades aged under 10 years. For all other age groups and grades the rates appear to have increased, although for the lowest grades over 20 years the increase is very small. The American figures quoted above also show that the decline in rates for those aged 10–14 applied only to high grade patients, and similarly show a decline for high-grade patients aged 5–9 (although an increase for those under this age). The fall in American admission rates for patients aged over 15 years applied mainly to the high-grade. But it is interesting that the rates for the high-grade aged 15–19 were, during the periods covered, only about half as great as those for the same group in England and Wales, and the rates for those over this age were only a fraction of the England and Wales figures. In general, during the periods covered by Sabagh and Windle, the rates of admission for idiots were higher, and for imbeciles and feeble-minded patients lower, than in this country during the later periods. The grade/age *pattern*, however, was substantially the same.

The highest rates of admission in both periods are for feeble-minded patients aged 15–19 years. It has been shown for the Manchester Region that about half of the male patients in this age group are admitted through the courts and half the females because they were said to be 'in moral danger' (Leeson, 1963). It would be useful to know whether this is true generally, and also for what reasons the remaining half are admitted.

If the increase in admissions over 35 years was confined only to *numbers*, this could be accounted for by the fact that there was an increase in the number of people in this age group in the home population. However, this would not account for the increased *rates* of admission for this age group. The increase in admission rates for the over-35s since 1949–51 is greater, proportionately, than for any other age group and applies to all three grades.

In so far as these figures are valid, it appears that, between 1949 and 1960, there was only one patient group for whom hospital admission was declining, i.e. the feeble-minded under the age of 16. These patients may have benefited from the increasing improvement in community services during these years, which obviated the need for admission. Alternatively they may have been rejected for admission to hospital mainly because of the more urgent needs of other patients.

TRAINING AND EDUCATION OF INPATIENTS

At the time the study was carried out no national figures were published showing the number of patients in hospital receiving training, and indeed these did not appear until 1970. It is perhaps indicative of the way that the hospital service has been viewed up to the present date that previously no routine figures were collected from hospitals on schooling work or training facilities, although local authorities were required to make such returns annually. The D.H.S.S. Statistical Report Series (No. 10) shows that, in 1964, 54 per cent of patients under the age of 16 were receiving education of some kind, and a rather larger percentage of adults are stated to be in education or employed or occupied in some way, either within or outside the hospital grounds. An analysis is given of the reasons why the remaining patients were not participating in these activities. This suggests that only 3 per cent of children and 5 per cent of adults were idle due to lack of facilities. Figures given in another table in the same publication show that there are marked variations between hospital regions in the ratio of instructors and teachers available, and it seems unlikely that this reflects real differences in the proportion of trainable patients in residence. In the light of the research reported in the following two chapters and the discussion by Pauline Morris of the paucity of education and training facilities in the hospitals she studied, one wonders what criterion hospitals used to define occupation or to judge the capacity to participate in it. Kushlick's studies in Wessex reveal that only one-third of adult patients are in formal training or education but over 55 per cent of residents are completely independent and without behaviour disorders. It seems unlikely that the facilities for employing patients in the Wessex Region are radically different from those in the rest of the country.

CONCLUSION

Well over half of the mentally handicapped population now lives in the community, and for most of those aged under 16 years some kind of training is provided by the Local Authorities. Only one third of patients over this age are receiving training. For an unknown number of recognized patients living in the community some kind of supervision is provided by visits from the staff of the Social Service Departments of the Local Authorities. In addition, a very small proportion are provided with residential accommodation in the community.

The remainder of handicapped patients are in hospitals administered by the Regional Hospital Boards. Figures published by the Ministry of Health and the Registrar General for the number of subnormal patients resident in hospitals show an increase between 1949 and 1959 of approximately 6,000 patients, that is, an increase of nearly 10 per cent. It seems likely that a further increase in residents has occurred since 1959, but the extent of the increase is difficult to estimate because of administrative changes and differences in the way statistics have been collected as a result.

Between 1949 and 1960 admissions, discharges and deaths for hospitals for the mentally retarded were increasing overall. Further analysis suggests that towards the end of the period the numbers of high-grade patients in hospitals were falling, while the numbers of low-grade patients were increasing, and this supports the findings on changes in the hospital population revealed by localized research studies. The greatest increase, both in numbers and rates of admissions, occurred amongst patients aged over 35 years.

Between 1960 and 1963 there was apparently an overall steep increase both in numbers and rates of admission, followed by a slower rise to 1967, but this apparent increase is difficult to interpret. Some of the change is doubtless due to a real increase in admissions, as a result of an increased turnover of patients, and in particular because of the rapid growth in short-stay care designed to give families a temporary relief. However it seems likely that in part the apparent rise in admissions is also due to administrative changes.

The changes from time to time in the definitions of terms used in collecting national statistics lessen their value as indicators of trends. However, even if the published figures are assumed to give a broadly accurate picture of what happened between 1948 and 1968, there clearly remain a number of key questions, summarized in our introductory chapter, which can be answered only by more detailed investigations.

3

A SURVEY OF HOSPITAL FACILITIES

In the previous chapters we showed how incomplete was the existing information, at a national level, on the characteristics of the hospital population. Knowledge of this kind is an essential element in any assessment of the adequacy of services, and with this in mind we sent, in July 1965, a questionnaire to all hospitals for the mentally handicapped in England and Wales administered by Regional Hospital Boards. This asked for information about the sex, grade and age (under 16 years and 16 years and over) of all resident patients at the end of 1964. Questions were also included about the numbers of patients in schools or training centres, and numbers working, as well as about the provision of other facilities. Among other purposes the survey was intended to provide comparative information for the more detailed study of residents in three Regions described in the next chapter.

All but three of the hospitals to which we wrote returned a questionnaire, but the returns made by a number of the participating hospitals were insufficiently complete for some of the analyses we undertook. The returns we received covered 85 per cent of the resident population. More particularly they covered 97 per cent of patients resident in hospitals for the mentally handicapped administered by Regional Hospital Boards – the population we sought to delineate.

CHARACTERISTICS OF HOSPITAL POPULATION

Eighty-six per cent of 53,272 patients were aged 16 years or over. This percentage is precisely reflected in the three Regions selected for more detailed study and reported on in the following chapter. The percentage of adults, that is people aged 16 years or over, varied between Regions from 70 to 95 per cent. But if we group together two Regions which shared facilities and

TABLE 3.1

AGE AND SEX OF PATIENTS RESIDENT IN HOSPITAL BY REGIONS

Region	Under 16 years Total patients	Males %	Over 16 years Total patients	Males %	Total	% under 16
1	713	45	2,176	51	2,889	25
2	571	63	3,483	48	4,054	14
3	267	60	936	60	1,203	22
4	564	5	3,718	56	4,282	13*
5	1,071	63	5,627	55	6,698	16*
6	463	64	4,370	56	4,833	10
7	288	64	1,519	46	1,807	16*
8	374	56	2,297	50	2,671	14*
9	601	57	4,766	52	5,367	11*
10	323	65	5,740	58	6,063	5
11	174	38	695	26	869	20
12	587	63	3,288	56	3,875	16*
13	162	56	1,332	54	1,494	11*
14	734	50	4,919	34	5,653	17*
15	449	61	1,065	42	1,514	30*
TOTAL	7,341	57	45,931	51	53,272	14
Grouped Regions 10 and 15	772	62	6,805	56	7,577	10

Notes: (a) * Complete Regions, i.e. Regions where every hospital surveyed co-operated in the inquiry.

(b) Patients in hospitals making a return with no classification by age = 2,339.

(c) Grouped Regions. Regions 10 and 15 shared hospital facilities, and it is therefore more sensible to consider them as one Region from some aspects, particularly age.[1]

(d) The Region numbers given here are not the numbers usually assigned to Regions in the Department of Health publications, since some Regions wished their material to remain confidential.

[1] The return for one of these Regions (No. 10) is incomplete. About 160 patients are missing. If all these patients were aged less than 16 years, the percentage for this Region would be seven rather than five, but if they were all aged 16 years or more the percentage of under 16s would remain at five.

consider only those Regions returning questionnaires for all their hospitals, the range of variation is narrowed to from 83 to 90 per cent. This is shown in Table 3.1 together with details of sex. Our results are similar to the figures derived from the Ministry of Health's Annual Report for 1964.

The variations in sex composition between Regions appear at first to be considerable but, again, if those sharing facilities are pooled the fluctuations are not so great. Thus the proportion of males among all patients aged less than 16 years ranges from 56 to 65 per cent and between 48 and 56 per cent for those aged 16 years and over. The one complete Region which turns out to have a lower proportion of males than females in hospital presents a surprising picture, both because it is accepted that mental handicap is more prevalent among males than females, and because there is reason to believe that hospital admission is more frequently sought for mentally handicapped males.

The figures relating to the grade of patients in hospital proved to be suspect for three reasons. First, unlike the figures for age and sex, there was very wide variation between Regions. This is not confirmed by other studies (Primrose, 1966) or by our own ward study (Chapter 4). Secondly when the data for all Regions were combined the proportion of low-grade patients in the hospital appeared to be considerably greater than would have been predicted on the basis of other enquiries. And, thirdly, a comparison of the figures obtained by this method with those elicited by a more intensive study of three Regions – an enquiry described in Chapter 4 – also revealed a considerable over-estimate of low-grade patients in the postal enquiry.

That the reported distribution of grades of defect should be inaccurate is not surprising, since experience suggests that, in general, record systems in hospitals for the mentally handicapped are not designed to enable the characteristics of the resident population to be readily and rapidly assessed. Answers to the kind of questions we asked are, therefore, almost invariably based on rough estimates.[2]

---

[2] At least one hospital searched individual records to ensure that the figures on grading were accurate in as far as the original assignment of grade was correct, but we know that in other cases this was not done. Fairly accurate estimates of sex and age groups of patients are more easily arrived at because men and women, children and adults are usually housed in different wards.

EMPLOYMENT AND TRAINING OF PATIENTS

Hospitals were asked to state how many patients were receiving training or schooling, how many were engaged on industrial contract work, how many received occupational therapy and how many went out to work each day.

Children, aged under 16 years

For the purposes of this and the following section, patients are divided into low-grade (I.Q. less than 25 approx.) and higher-grade (I.Q. 25 and over). This dichotomy, rather than the conventional one distinguishing between I.Q. under and over 50 is used because it is more relevant to the provision of training and occupation. The figures for grading obtained from the hospital questionnaire have not been used, for the reasons already given. Instead we have used the proportions indicated by the ward study (Chapter 4) of roughly one-third low-grade and two-thirds higher-grade – proportions consistent with other recent studies of residents (Primrose, 1966; Kushlick, 1969).

The figures of children attending school are likely to be more or less accurate because they are easily ascertained and would in the normal course of events be known to the hospital administration. There is reasonable agreement, for the three Regions described in the ward study, between the two surveys (hospital survey 44 per cent of under 16s at school : ward study 40 per cent), and the national figure for the hospital survey is similar to that shown for a national sample of hospitals investigated by Morris (1969).

Table 3.2 shows the percentage of children in hospital attending a school or training centre and compares this with the percentage estimated to be of higher grade. If only the higher-grade patients are assumed to be eligible for training, 28 per cent of these patients in England and Wales are shown not to be receiving training, and the proportion varies from 1 per cent to 59 per cent between Regions. It can be argued that the estimated proportion of higher-grade patients is inaccurate for incomplete Regions. If only complete Regions are considered the proportion remaining untrained still varies from 10 per cent to 44 per cent (two Regions pooled).

Some of the higher-grade children not attending school may be handicapped in ways which make training difficult in present

TABLE 3.2

PATIENTS UNDER 16 YEARS OF AGE ATTENDING SCHOOL OR
TRAINING-CENTRE, AS PERCENTAGE OF ESTIMATED NUMBERS OF
HIGHER-GRADE PATIENTS

Region	Total children (under 16 yrs)	Est. higher-grade = ⅔ of total (from ward study)	No. at school	No. at school as % of estimated nos. of higher-grade pts
1	607	405	320	79
2	442	295	178	60
3	267	178	126	71
4	564*	376	245	65*
5	1,071*	714	593	84*
6	463	309	243	79
7	153	102	77	64
8	374*	251	169	67*
9	601*	401	360	90*
10	323	215	212	99
11	174	116	48	41
12	587*	392	267	69*
13	162*	108	60	56*
14	564	376	248	66
15	449*	299	125	42*
TOTAL	6,801	4,537	3,273	72
Grouped Regions 10 and 15	772	515	337	65

Notes: (a) * Complete Regions, i.e. covering all patients in the hospitals surveyed in that Region.

(b) Grouped Regions. Regions 10 and 15 shared hospital facilities and it is therefore more sensible to consider them as one Region from some aspects.

circumstances. The ward study shows that 23 per cent of higher-grade children were either under 5 years old or handicapped in some way (although only 15 per cent had severe educational handicaps, i.e. blind or unable to use their hands). However, the proportion of severely disabled high-grade patients is unlikely to vary as greatly between Regions as the proportion shown to be receiving schooling, and we suggest that at least ten Regions are providing fewer opportunities for training for child patients than are required. These are the ten Regions providing schooling for less than 75 per cent of the estimated number of higher-grade patients.

It may be helpful to consider the foregoing figures against the background of the answers given to our question concerning the availability of schools and junior training centres. Only five hospitals out of seventy-three claiming to house medium- or high-grade children had no school. In all but one of these the number of children involved was fewer than ten. On the other hand, twelve out of fifteen hospitals claiming to house only or mainly low-grade children (338 patients) provided no school. This is acceptable if all these children have in fact an I.Q. of less than 25. However, since we have reason to believe that there has been an over-estimate of the number of low-grade patients, it is quite possible that some of these children could benefit from training. Of the total of seventeen hospitals (housing 435 patients) which provided no school, seven (265 patients) said that their patients were severely handicapped, one was described as a nursery unit (19 patients), and one (24 patients) sent a single patient to a local training centre, suggesting that facilities were available if needed. None of the seventeen hospitals said that they were in need of a school. Only a more intensive study could show whether or not any of the patients involved were being deprived of training from which they could benefit, but in view of the number of children involved some further investigation is surely necessary.

Adults, aged 16 years or over
Table 3.3 shows the percentage of patients aged 16 years and over who were occupied in one of four ways (i.e. industrial contract work, outside employment, training and occupational therapy), and compares this with the percentage shown by the ward study to be of medium or high grade. Over half of the higher-grade adults were unoccupied in one of the ways mentioned; if the more purposive employment on industrial contract work, outside employment or training is considered, only just over one-sixth are so occupied. In the ward study only 27 per cent of higher-grade adults were found to be over the age of 65 or severely handicapped (that is blind or unable to use their hands) and who might not, therefore, be expected to work. On this basis, about one-third of capable adult patients were not occupied in one of these ways, and about three-quarters were not purposively occupied.

The proportions of patients working or training are almost

TABLE 3.3

PATIENTS AGED 16 YEARS AND OVER OCCUPIED IN FOUR WAYS COMPARED WITH THE ESTIMATED NUMBER OF HIGHER-GRADE PATIENTS

Region	Total patients aged over 16 years	Estimated number of higher-grade patients = 90% of total patients (from ward study)	(a) Number in industrial contract work	(b) Number going out to work	(c) Number at school	(d) Number in occupational therapy	Total working or at school as % of estimated higher-grade patients	Total working at school, or in occupational therapy as % of estimated higher-grade patients
1	1,601	1,441	15	48	34	539	6	44
2	3,143	2,829	292	86	98	489	15	34
3	936	842	183	17	43	155	26	47
4*	3,718	3,346	251	147	1	1,703	11*	63*
5*	5,627	5,064	929	291	79	603	23*	38*
6	4,370	3,933	506	301	140	1,227	22	55
7	798	768	132	119	1	151	32	56
8*	2,297	2,067	245	42	70	483	16*	41*
9*	4,766	4,289	523	229	38	797	17*	37*
10	5,740	5,166	754	100	104	1,357	17	45
11	695	626	101	41	39	44	26	36
12	3,000	2,700	87	108	34	919	8	43
13*	1,332	1,199	66	58	55	325	13*	42*
14	3,445	3,101	496	76	25	236	17	27
15*	1,065	959	120	28	57	376	19*	61*
TOTAL	42,533	38,280	4,700	1,691	818	9,404	17	43

* Complete Regions.

identical with those found by Morris, but two points should be made about the totals of patients occupied shown by this survey. First, we did not ask for the number of patients working about the hospital, and therefore it cannot be assumed that all those patients who were not employed in one of the ways mentioned were wholly unemployed. Secondly, we did not attempt a definition of occupational therapy, and it is by no means certain that all the patients said to be in occupational therapy were better employed than those helping with the maintenance of the hospital (although in a few cases patients working in service departments of the hospital, e.g. shoe repairing, were included as O.T. patients).

When the questionnaire was drafted we had in mind the kind of employment which is designed primarily for the patient's benefit, whether as a means of returning him to the community or as a meaningful way of occupying his life. At the time the occupations chosen appeared to fulfil this criterion, but subsequent discussions with hospital staff suggest that useful work in the hospital – for example, sweeping floors, or helping to look after a younger and more handicapped patient – could, *if it is planned*, be a more effective form of rehabilitation or means of preventing institutionalization than traditional occupational therapy (e.g. basket-weaving). The arguments against the employment of patients on maintenance and domestic work are that it is at present largely designed to make good a shortage of staff and not to rehabilitate patients, and that it may in fact even discourage the discharge of patients who are useful to the hospital. It may also conceal the shortage of staff which, if available, might help the patient towards independence more effectively. The whole question of employment and occupation for the mentally handicapped both in hospitals and in the community obviously needs careful reappraisal.

It is not possible to derive from this postal survey a precise estimate of the extent to which patients in hospital lack adequate employment, but it is clear that about 80 per cent of higher-grade patients were occupied in ways which neither were geared to returning them to the community nor provided sheltered workshop conditions. Some 27 per cent of the same patients may have been too old or too handicapped to work, but again only more intensive studies could reveal how many of the remaining 50 per cent were well occupied.

Most hospitals reported that they provided some industrial contract work, or had arrangements for sending patients out to work, however small the number involved. However twenty-four hospitals with higher-grade patients had no workshop and sent no patients out to work; this involved 1,176 higher-grade patients, who were mostly concentrated in two Regions. Of these twenty-four hospitals, three were probably geriatric units (56 patients), one was providing active psychiatric treatment for disturbed patients, not yet ready for occupation (17 patients), and one was employing female patients as domestics as part of a rehabilitation scheme (4 patients). Of the remaining nineteen hospitals, three said they were in need of occupational facilities and two claimed that the present accommodation was quite unsuitable. All but five (57 patients)[3] of the hospitals with higher-grade patients and lacking industrial contract work or arrangements for patients to work outside the hospital, provided occupational therapy and their patients should not necessarily be assumed to be less well occupied. Some contract work certainly requires less skill than some O.T. work, and patients in a workshop may spend much of their time doing nothing if proper conditions of employment are not encouraged. Nevertheless it is probably true that a good workshop is more likely to help in training a patient for community life than good occupational therapy. Equally, a hospital providing even inadequate contract work is more likely to be aware of the aim of returning patients to the outside world wherever possible than a hospital providing occupational therapy only.

Of course for many, if not most, patients full return to the community is necessarily an impracticable aim, and the type of occupation suitable for them has to be decided on grounds other than its relevance to outside employment, although even for these patients a good workshop may produce a high level of work satisfaction. Certainly it should be established that they are being adequately occupied in some way.

OTHER HOSPITAL ACTIVITIES

In addition to answering questions about training and industrial facilities, the hospitals were asked about the provision of

[3] Of these 57 patients 23 were geriatric and one was blind.

certain special services, about co-operation with local authorities and about additional provisions which they considered necessary.

Seventy-seven out of 123 hospitals with higher-grade adults claimed that a member of hospital staff was responsible for finding work for patients, and seventy said that it was the responsibility of someone in the hospital to find accommodation for patients when necessary. Only forty-two hospitals, however, mentioned a social worker as being responsible for each task. It may be that a hostel warden (mentioned by seven hospitals) is as effective as a social worker in finding employment and accommodation, but it is unlikely that a matron, medical superintendent, or assistant chief male nurse, mentioned by the remaining hospitals, would have the same time or specialist knowledge to devote to these tasks as would a social worker. Some hospitals maintained that one or both of these tasks was the duty of the Mental Welfare Officers of the Local Health Authority. But in this case the effectiveness of the arrangements would depend upon the relationship between the hospital and the L.H.A.

Hospitals were in fact asked whether they co-operated with the Local Health Authority. Sixty-eight out of 126 hospitals replied that they did so, but only fifty gave actual examples of liaison. Examples given referred to the interchange of training facilities.

The forms of co-operation between the hospitals and Local Authorities are shown below.

Form of Co-operation	No. of Hospitals
Day patients (purpose unspecified)	12
Day patients received for training centre or workshop	10
Hospital Patients to L.H.A. training centre and workshop	9
Joint training centre provided by hospital and L.H.A.	2
Hospital Patients sent to L.E.A. school	5
L.E.A. provide evening classes for hospital patients	14
L.E.A. provide teachers for unspecified classes	2
Hospital patients attend L.H.A. social club	3
Mental welfare officers co-operate with or act as hospital social workers	7
Medical Superintendent sits on L.H.A. committee or acts as L.H.A. consultant	4
Joint case conferences between L.H.A. and hospital staff	3

Form of Co-operation	No. of Hospitals
Liaison committee exists, or joint mental health service	4
Other	4

Twenty Hospitals mentioned more than one form of liaison.

Of those twenty-two hospitals which received day patients from the community, three said they took specially selected patients (e.g. those who were too disturbed to be acceptable in an L.H.A. training centre) and two said they took community patients pending the provision of a training centre by the Local Authority. The former case seems sensible, but in the latter the phrase 'pending provision etc.' emphasizes the division existing at present between hospital and community patients. The mixing of the two kinds of patients is seen as a temporary arrangement rather than as a means of integrating the hospital patient into the community. The most useful example of co-operation in training from the point of view of rehabilitation may well be the cases where hospital patients are sent to Local Authority training-centres and workshops.

Only fourteen hospitals said they co-operated with the Local Education Authority in the provision of evening classes (although there were altogether fifty hospitals out of 123 with higher-grade adult patients which provided evening classes). In view of the finding of the British Psychological Society (1966) that 14 per cent of testable children admitted to hospital in 1961 had I.Q.s of over 70, the number of hospitals co-operating with Local Education Authorities, other than for evening classes, appears small. The education of children in this I.Q. range has always been in fact the responsibility of the Education Authorities, although in some cases patients' behaviour disorders may complicate provision.[4]

Finally, hospitals were asked what amenities they lacked and would like to see introduced. Their answers should obviously not be interpreted as providing a quantitative measure of facilities which are lacking. When asked an open question about gaps in services, people (including hospital administrators) are not always able to recall all the deficiencies

[4] Since the time of this enquiry the responsibility for the education of all children has been accepted by the Department of Education and Science.

they experience; nor for that matter may they really be aware of them. Only six hospitals, for instance, said they needed more nursing staff, although this need must be common to the great majority of hospitals. Furthermore, the questionnaire up to this point had concentrated on training and occupational activities, and the need for an improvement of these was predictably mentioned frequently. However, the items recorded do give a useful indication of the range of provisions which are manifestly lacking, and are therefore summarized in the following table.

Reported Need	No. of Hospitals
Extension of employment or occupational facilities	29
More or improved accommodation	18
Extension or improvement of educational facilities	17
Physiotherapist, or more physiotherapists	12
Swimming-pool	12
Psychologist, or more psychologists	10
Hostel, or more hostels	10
Diagnostic or assessment unit	9
Laboratory and staff	6
More nursing staff	6
More or improved staff accommodation	6
Children's unit (small, family type of unit)	6
Socialization unit	6
Evening classes, or more evening classes	5
Speech therapist	5
Disturbed or security unit	5
Geriatric accommodation	5
Domestic science training	5
Special care unit (unspecified)	5
Other (items mentioned four times or less)	30

CONCLUSION

Seventeen hospitals having children provided no school or training centre; for nine of these hospitals a school was probably inappropriate, but for the remaining eight the situation is unclear. Since our questionnaires covered a different number of units for each hospital, it is not certain that the children in these eight hospitals were worse off than others who may be situated, for example, in outlying buildings of larger hospitals which possess one school for patients in the main building only. However, it is a cause for concern that such a low proportion of children are attending schools in many Regions – 40 per cent overall, or 72 per cent of higher-grade children. The important question is not so much whether hospitals have schools or not, but whether all the children who are capable of being trained are able to attend a school or a training centre, either within the hospital or elsewhere, and whether the provision of school staff and accommodation are adequate. The evidence reviewed in this chapter suggests that at least at the time of this enquiry, they were not.

It cannot be said from this survey how far adults were under-occupied. Very few of the higher-grade patients were employed in ways related to life outside hospitals. Only five hospitals provided nothing in the way of industrial contract work, outside employment or occupational therapy. It would seem that few hospitals provided sufficient employment, and this impression is confirmed by the study described in the next chapter.

Perhaps the most interesting finding here is the fact that hospital administrators, who willingly returned a questionnaire and clearly wished to cooperate in this study, were very often unable to answer accurately simple questions regarding the characteristics of hospital residents. The hospital survey reported in this chapter is intended only as a first step in the delineation of need, and the precise location of deficiencies is a task best carried out at a ward level. In the next chapter the results of one method of approaching the problem are described.

In conclusion it should be recognized that many authorities are aware of the deficiencies of their services. This is not especially true of the individual hospitals in their replies to our questionnaire, where it is the range of additional facilities desired rather than the recognition of deficits which is of interest. The Regional Boards did seem to be more aware of poor provision, and in several cases pointed out to us that they knew the present service was inadequate and that plans existed, or were in process of implementation, for the improvement of existing conditions.

4

CAPACITIES AND HANDICAPS OF
HOSPITAL PATIENTS

In order to provide good residential services one needs to know details of the grade and age of the patients they house and of the patients' capacities to care for themselves and to work. The degree of independence they can achieve also depends upon the physical and behavioural handicaps from which they suffer, so that we must know about this too. The present study was an attempt to discover the characteristics of hospital in-patients with a view to assessing their training and nursing needs. In July 1965 questionnaires were sent to the nurses in charge of each ward in every N.H.S. hospital for the mentally handicapped in three of the fifteen hospital Regions. The Regions were not selected on a random basis but because they appeared to be very different from one another. One was a metropolitan and suburban area, one covered another conur-bation, and the third was almost entirely rural. It was hoped that by considering these three Regions we would cover the full range of problems encountered among hospitals for the mentally handicapped.

The nurses completing the questionnaire were asked to check a list of items for every tenth patient on the ward register. These items referred to the sex, age, grade, physical handicaps, behaviour problems and occupation of patients, and were described in terms found to be meaningful to the nursing staff concerned with their everyday care. Information on 1,080 patients was obtained in this way, representing a total of some 10,000 in the three Regions combined.

We decided that it was necessary to grade patients in some way equivalent to the threefold classification used up to 1959, since for a number of reasons this seemed the best one to use. Firstly, it was not practicable to ask for the patients' I.Q. since only a small proportion of patients have had an I.Q. test, and since intelligence quotients are not useful unless details of the particular test used and the age of the patient when tested are also available. Secondly, we decided that for this study the categories high-, medium- and low-grade could not be reliably applied, because these are inherently relative terms, and therefore 'high-grade' to a nurse working entirely with severely handicapped patients might mean something different compared with a nurse whose experience was confined to more intelligent patients. In practice we found that nurses were familiar with the older terminology, idiot, imbecile, feeble-minded, and were quite happy to use these categories, which, although out of fashion since the 1959 Act, do at least have the advantage of providing for a threefold classification with reasonably clear boundaries.[1]

SEX

Table 4.1 shows the age and sex structure of the inpatient population. In all three Regions the proportion of males exceeded that of female patients (males 56 per cent). This is a common finding for the mentally handicapped, both those in hospital (O'Connor and Tizard, 1954; Primrose, 1966), and those in the community (Lewis, 1929; Gruenberg, 1964). The community studies usually report the greatest excess of males in the youngest age groups and lowest grades (Gruenberg, 1964). In the present survey the excess of males over females was also found to be greatest in the younger age groups, and, indeed, over the age of 35 the sexes are almost equally represented. Unlike the community studies, however, the sex difference was found at all grades in about the same ratio.

AGE

Most official statistics summarize the age structure of subnormal populations by groups over and under 16. This is meaningful in administrative terms, since schooling for the educational subnormal and the mentally handicapped is usually provided only for those under 16 years, and Local Authority training

[1] Further details of this study and a copy of the questionnaire are contained in Appendix 2.

TABLE 4.1

AGE AND SEX OF RESIDENTS

Age in years	0–5	6–15	16–25	26–35	36–45	46–55	55–65	66–75	75+	Total	%
Male	5	69	134	95	80	103	72	36	6	600	56
Female	0	46	90	68	84	76	74	29	13	480	44
Total residents	5	115	224	163	164	179	146	65	19	1,080	100
Per cent	—	11	21	15	15	17	13	6	2	100	—

departments usually transfer patients at about 16 years from junior to adult training centres. However, this is not necessarily the most useful age at which to divide the mentally handicapped. By 16 years the mentally handicapped are still functioning intellectually at a level somewhere below that of the average twelve-year-old and there is no good reason to regard them as fully adult, except possibly in terms of physiological maturity. Intellectually and often emotionally also, they still require the treatment appropriate to a child of a much younger age, and there is ample evidence to show that they can still benefit greatly from training and education beyond the age of 16 years (Clarke, 1965) and can even improve in tested intelligence, given the correct type of stimulation.

In the present survey, therefore, we have divided patients into groups under and over 16 only to make comparison with other data, and have sometimes chosen instead to concentrate upon the division of the residential population into young persons and adults, defined as those of 25 years and less, and those of over 25 years. The decision to use 25 years as a cut-off point is perhaps arbitrary there being no data available on which to base a more rational decision. However, by this age most middle- and high-grade patients who might be candidates for discharge are functioning at a mental-age level somewhere between 12 and 16 years, and it is likely that, if by this age a patient is not regarded as fit for discharge, he will probably remain in some form of residential care indefinitely. There is some indirect evidence for this in that well over 80 per cent of the patients aged over 25 years have been in hospital for more than fifteen years. These patients, with little chance of returning fully to the community, are likely to require employment and occupation rather than education and training, and to this extent need a different kind of service from that given to the younger patients.

Table 4.1 shows that only 8 per cent of residents are aged over 65 years and that one-third are under 25 years of age, the largest group being aged from 16 to 25 years. Eleven per cent of residents are aged 15 or under, which, perhaps surprisingly, is about the same proportion as found in earlier studies (O'Connor and Tizard, 1954; Primrose, 1966). It is possible that the proportions of children and adults in hospital are very largely determined by the number of wards allocated to them and that, unless special new accommodation is built, the proportion of inpatients under and over 16 does not vary much over time regardless of need. Primrose (1966) showed that the absolute numbers of children admitted to a large hospital group in Scotland increased only as a result of extra accommodation being built.

GRADE RELATED TO AGE, AND TO AGE ON ADMISSION

Table 4.2 shows the number of patients of each grade sub-divided according to age. Twelve per cent of the total population are idiots. Over 70 per cent of these patients are 25 years or under, and less than 1 per cent are over 65. Most of them were admitted under the age of 10 years (see Table 4.3) and their present age distribution presumably results from this together with their low expectation of life.[2]

Imbeciles are by far the most numerous patients and form over half the hospital population (54 per cent). They are more evenly distributed amongst the age groups and just over one-third are aged 25 or less. Most of them were admitted to hospital under the age of 20, the majority between 11 and 20 years. Unlike the low-grade patients, however, a considerable proportion of them also came into hospital at later ages, and 20 per cent of them had been admitted over the age of 40 years.

A little over one-third of the resident population is feeble-minded. These are on average the oldest patients, and were admitted at the oldest ages. Only a quarter of feeble-minded patients are 25 years or under, while 11 per cent are over 65 years of age, and, unlike the lower grades, hardly any were admitted under the age of 10 years. As with imbeciles, there was a peak period of admission between 11 and 20 years, but nearly one-half came in between the ages of 21 and 40.

The grade structure of the hospital population in the three Regions is very different from that found by O'Connor and Tizard in London in 1952 (see Table 4.2) although very simi-

---

[2] There could be other explanations: for example, there may have been an increase in the numbers of young low-grade patients admitted in recent years, but this alternative is not likely. See Hospital Cohort Study, Chapter 5.

TABLE 4.2

NUMBER AND PERCENTAGE OF RESIDENTS IN EACH AGE AND GRADE GROUP

Age group	0–5	6–15	16–25	26–65	65+	Total	%	% 1952*
Idiot[1]	3	38	47	37	1	126	12	6
Imbecile	2	73	119	348	41	583	54	42
Feeble-minded	0	4	58	267	42	371	34	52
Total number of residents	5	115	224	652	84	1,080	100	100

Note: * Figures taken from O'Connor and Tizard, 1954.
[1] Percentages have been rounded up and consequently the percentages given in each cell in this group do not add up to 12 per cent.

TABLE 4.3

PERCENTAGE OF RESIDENTS ADMITTED IN DIFFERENT AGE GROUPS, FOR EACH OF THE THREE GRADES

Age on admission	0–10	11–20	21–40	41+	Total	%
Idiot	55	32	9	4	126	100
Imbecile	26	30	26	17	583	100
Feeble-minded	5	29	46	20	371	100
Total residents	236	324	338	182	1,080	
Per cent	22	30	31	17	100	

lar to what Primrose found in Scotland in 1964. The present study shows a much smaller percentage of feeble-minded patients, especially at the younger ages, than in O'Connor and Tizard's study (34 per cent compared with 52 per cent). Correspondingly there is a greater percentage of middle- and low-grade patients (66 per cent compared with 48 per cent), and in particular the proportion of idiots in the age groups over 16 years has increased greatly. The change in the percentage of high-grade patients actually occupying beds is not as great as appears from these figures, however, since 9 per cent of the patients included as residents in the 1952 study were actually on licence in the community.

LENGTH OF STAY

Over half the idiots had been in hospital for less than ten years, and only 13 per cent for more than twenty years (see Table

4.4). This is related to their age distribution, reflecting their comparatively short expectation of life, but it may to some extent be the result of increased numbers of admissions in recent years. By contrast, although over 40 per cent of imbecile and feeble-minded patients had been in hospital for less than ten years, nearly a third had been resident for twenty years or more.

TABLE 4.4

PERCENTAGE OF PATIENTS RESIDENT FOR DIFFERENT LENGTHS OF TIME, FOR EACH OF THE THREE GRADES

No. of years resident	0–5	6–10	11–20	21+	Total	%
Idiot	23	31	32	13	126	100
Imbecile	22	23	26	29	583	100
Feeble-minded	25	16	26	33	371	100
Total residents	251	232	290	307	1,080	
Per cent	23	21	27	28	100	

Looking at the population as a whole, over half of the residents had been in hospital for over ten years and nearly 30 per cent for over twenty years. Discharge rates for recently admitted patients have been rising at least since 1949, as will be shown in Chapter 6. But patients who have been in hospital for ten years or more are unlikely to be able to return to their homes in the community. Most of them will grow old and die in residential care of some kind. Nearly half of the most able patients, the feeble-minded, were over 45 at the time of this survey, and two-thirds of them had been in hospital for ten years or more. As they age they will be less capable of helping with the domestic duties of the hospital, as some of them have done in the past. Nevertheless they will still require occupation of some kind, even though this cannot be geared to their return to the community.

PHYSICAL HANDICAP

Table 4.5 shows the incidence of physical and sensory handicap among inpatients. A patient is counted as having a physical handicap if he cannot walk unaided, cannot use one or both hands normally, is epileptic, blind or deaf.[3] Thirty-seven per cent of patients suffer from one of these disabilities, and 12 per cent of all patients have multiple handicaps.[4]

The prevalence of handicap and multiple handicap is closely related to grade, as can be seen in Table 4.5. This is not altogether surprising since low-grade patients are known to suffer from a high incidence of brain damage and physical handicap. However, one might have expected to find a greater prevalence of handicap among the feeble-minded to account for their admission to hospital. The distribution of handicap also varies with age, and while nearly half of those under 25 suffer from some handicap, only one-third of those over 25 do so. This is

TABLE 4.5

PERCENTAGE OF PATIENTS IN EACH GRADE AND AGE GROUP WITH SOME PHYSICAL HANDICAP

Age in years	0–15	16–25	26–65	66+	Total	%
Idiot total	41	47	37	1	126	100
% Any handicaps	61	79	51	100	82	65
% Multiple handicaps	34	21	13	—	29	23
Imbecile total	75	119	348	41	583	100
% Any handicaps	44	39	34	39	214	37
% Multiple handicaps	13	15	12	17	78	13
Feeble-minded total	4	58	267	42	371	100
% Any handicaps	25	19	29	31	102	28
% Multiple handicaps	25	5	7	12	29	8
Total residents	120	224	652	84	1,080	100
% Any handicaps	49	42	33	36	398	37
% Multiple handicaps	21	14	10	14	136	12

[3] We preferred to use these behavioural measures of handicap rather than to ask for specific diagnoses, for example cerebral palsy, (a) because we thought it likely that nurses could be more precise about the former than the latter, (b) because much of the handicap among the mentally subnormal cannot readily be gathered under any diagnostic umbrella, and (c) because we were not in any case interested in the milder forms of handicap which would not interfere greatly with normal life, for example a cerebral-palsied patient with only a slight limp.

[4] These figures include those idiots who cannot walk alone, although this may represent a general learning deficit rather than a motor handicap.

probably because of the known higher mortality rate of young, low-grade patients, who are the ones most likely to have physical defects.

Motor handicap

Table 4.6 shows the percentage by grade of those who have a motor handicap, i.e. who are bedfast or who need help with walking or who cannot use one or both hands, and again this is closely related to grade. The percentage of the total population who cannot walk at all is very small, only 9 per cent, although in the idiot grade this rises to over one-third. Again while only 24 per cent of the total population are either bed-

TABLE 4.6

NUMBER AND PERCENTAGE OF PATIENTS IN EACH GRADE AND AGE
GROUP WITH A MOTOR HANDICAP, BY DEGREE OF DISABILITY

Age in years	6–15	16–25	26–65	66+	Total	%
Idiot total	41	47	31	1	126	100
Bedfast	17	20	8	1	46	36
Needs help walking	7	4	4	0	15	12
Crippled hands	15	19	6	1	41	32
Any motor handicap	24	27	16	1	68	54
Imbecile total	75	119	348	41	583	100
Bedfast	8	9	19	2	38	6
Needs help walking	6	5	24	3	38	6
Crippled hands	9	17	44	5	75	13
Any motor handicap	16	24	64	7	111	19
Feeble-minded total	4	58	267	42	371	100
Bedfast	0	2	7	4	13	3
Needs help walking	1	1	11	0	13	3
Crippled hands	1	1	25	3	30	8
Any motor handicap	1	4	39	6	50	13
Total residents	120	224	652	84	1,080	100
% Bedfast	21	14	5	8	99	9
% Needs help walking	12	4	6	4	163	15
% Crippled hands	19	16	11	11	149	14
% Any other handicap	34	25	18	17	229	21

fast or need help with walking, nearly half of all idiots have some difficulty with walking.

There is also a relationship between age and motor handicap, which is largely due to the concentration of idiots in the younger groups. The number of imbecile and feeble-minded patients who are handicapped are more evenly distributed over the age groups, but the proportions are always highest among the younger patients.

Epilepsy

Table 4.7 shows the distribution of epilepsy by age and grade. About 20 per cent of the total population is epileptic. In the present study a patient was counted as epileptic if he suffered from fits or was being treated with anti-convulsant drugs. About 63 per cent of those on drugs had actually had one or more epileptic fits in the previous twelve months.

Again there is a strong relationship between grade and epilepsy. The percentage of patients suffering from epilepsy

TABLE 4.7

PERCENTAGE OF PATIENTS IN EACH GRADE AND AGE GROUP WITH A
SENSORY HANDICAP OR EPILEPSY

Age in years	0–15	16–25	26–65	66+	Total	%
Idiot total	41	47	37	1	126	100
% Sensory defect	9	3	7	0	19	15
% Epilepsy	19	26	12	0	57	45
Imbecile total	75	119	348	41	583	100
% Sensory defect	6	8	21	10	45	8
% Epilepsy	16	28	64	5	113	19
Feeble-minded total	4	58	267	42	371	100
% Sensory defect	1	3	13	7	24	6
% Epilepsy	0	7	41	4	52	14
Total residents	120	224	652	84	1,080	100
% Sensory defect	13	6	6	20	88	8
% Epilepsy	29	27	18	11	222	20
% Deaf	2	3	3	18	41	4
% Blind	12	5	4	5	56	5

drops at older ages, partly because fewer idiots survive to middle age, but even in the two higher grades the prevalence of epilepsy is much lower in those over the age of 45.

Sensory defect

Only 4 per cent of the total population is said to be deaf (see Table 4.7). This figure is probably lower than the actual number with impaired hearing because nurses were told not to count a patient as deaf if he wore a hearing aid and could hear normally with it. However the number of mentally handicapped inpatients with hearing aids is likely to be fairly small.

The prevalence of reported deafness is fairly constant at all ages (about 2·5 per cent), until the age of 65, when it rises to 18 per cent. A number of facts suggest, however, that nurses tend to underestimate deafness among subnormals. Only one idiot is described as being deaf, although the true prevalence of deafness among low-grade patients must be much higher than this. No deafness was noted among the under tens, but again this seems hardly credible. The prevalence of deafness in the imbecile and feeble-minded grades is very similar, about 4 per cent for each, although the distribution of other physical handicaps suggests that deafness should be more common among imbeciles.

It seems possible that unless a patient is old enough and sufficiently high-grade to attempt a conversation, deafness is unlikely to be identified by the nursing staff. On the other hand, Hilliard and Kirman (1966) report a similar rate of deafness (3·5 per cent) in a population probably containing more low-grade patients than in our sample. There is an obvious need here for more detailed audiometric investigations.

A patient in this study is classified as 'blind or nearly blind' if the nursing staff judged him unable to see to pick up objects the size of a spoon. It is detected much more frequently than deafness, especially in the younger age groups. Other studies have also found that a visual impairment is a complaint more frequently registered than an auditory one, particularly for the youngest age groups (Tarjan, *et al.*, 1960). But there still may be some under-reporting in our figures, since Hilliard and Kirman (1966) quote an overall rate of 14 per cent whilst in the present study the overall incidence of blindness is only 5 per cent.

Again there is a relationship between age and defect, largely because of the greater numbers of idiots in the younger age groups. Ten per cent of those under 16 are blind, but nearly two-thirds of these are idiots. Nearly half of all blind patients under 25 years are idiots.

The figures given for blindness and deafness represent only the most severe type of sensory defect, i.e. almost total loss of vision or hearing, because it was not considered possible to get reliable estimates of milder forms of sensory impairment. There will be many patients in addition, therefore, whose capacities for learning and for independence are impaired by some degree of sensory defect which might be alleviated by mechanical aids. Much of this probably goes undiagnosed at the present time because these patients cannot communicate their problems easily, and the staff and facilities necessary to diagnose and treat do not exist in subnormality hospitals at present (Morris, 1969).

BEHAVIOUR

Although training and mechanical aids may improve a patient's capacity to learn and become independent, the relationship between his mental abilities and his performance is limited not only by his physical handicaps but also by any disturbance in behaviour or any mental illness that he shows.

Table 4.8 shows the distribution of behaviour disorders by age and grade and sex. Forty-three per cent of the hospital population in the three Regions showed some disorder. These were most common amongst the lowest-grade patients of whom 67 per cent were affected, and least common amongst the feeble-minded where they occurred in about one-quarter of the patients.

Table 4.9 shows the relationship between grade and the frequency of each disorder recorded. Withdrawal is the behaviour disorder most frequently reported and occurs in almost 20 per cent of the population. Some patients described as withdrawn may actually suffer from autism, i.e. a psychotic condition with poverty of language and bizarre behaviour being the most prominent symptoms. However, this is a fairly

TABLE 4.8

PERCENTAGE OF PATIENTS IN EACH GRADE AND AGE GROUP WITH A
BEHAVIOUR DISORDER

Age in years	0–15	16–25	26–45	46+	Total	%
Idiot total	41	47	22	16	126	100
% Single	54	79	68	69	85	67
% Multiple	29	38	50	37	47	37
Imbecile total	75	119	182	207	583	100
% Single	61	54	50	36	276	47
% Multiple	37	29	19	12	122	21
Feeble-minded total	4	58	123	186	371	100
% Single	50	48	28	20	102	37
% Multiple	25	26	7	6	36	10
Total residents	120	224	327	409	1,080	100
% Single	58	58	43	30	463	43
% Multiple	34	30	17	10	205	19

TABLE 4.9

PERCENTAGE OF PATIENTS IN EACH OF THE THREE GRADES SHOWING
EACH TYPE OF BEHAVIOUR DISORDER

Type of disorders	Idiot 126 = 100%	Imbecile 583 = 100%	Feeble-minded 371 = 100%	Total 1,080 = 100%
Withdrawal	29	20	10	18
Aggressive	17	20	12	17
Destructive	29	15	4	13
Hyperactivity	29	14	6	13
Attention-seeking	13	11	9	11
Self-injury	21	8	1	8
Percentage of residents tranquillized	38	24	18	24
Percentage of residents on Night sedation	17	10	6	10

rare condition even among hospital patients (Lotte, V., 1967), and most of the withdrawal noted here will be of a much less severe nature. Withdrawal is most common among low-grade patients, and this may simply mean that the patient is too retarded to take part in activities. However even if idiot patients are excluded, it remains the second most frequent disorder reported.

Aggression is the disorder next most frequently reported although in no group does it occur in more than 20 per cent of cases. It is the most common disorder among imbeciles and the feeble-minded, although more idiots than high-grade patients are aggressive. Destruction and hyperactivity are also common, and these are especially frequent among idiots. Attention-seeking is shown by all grades in roughly the same proportion, while self-injury is rare among the feeble-minded and is associated more with the lower grades, particularly idiots, of whom one-fifth are involved.

Behaviour disorders are least commonly reported among the feeble-minded, and multiple disorders are rare. Although it is possible that nurses view a particular activity in low-grade patients as a disturbance, while accepting it as normal in a higher-grade patient, this seems unlikely to account for the entire difference. Clearly it is improbable that what is considered as aggression, withdrawal etc in low-grade patients will constitute the same kind of activity receiving this description in the feeble-minded, since the repertoire of behaviour in each grade will be very different. For this reason a comparison of the distribution of particular disorders in different grades may not be valid. It may be, for example, that a low-grade patient who is withdrawn *and* destructive causes less disturbance in the ward than a high-grade patient who is destructive only; while a low-grade patient who persistently engages in self-assault, apparently without cause or motive, may be a much greater problem than a high-grade patient who occasionally makes a suicide attempt.

It is perhaps surprising to find that only just over a quarter of feeble-minded patients have behaviour disorders, as it is usually thought that this is a major cause of admission to hospital for these patients. It is possible that the kind of behaviour which often results in admissions cannot occur or is simply not provoked in the normal hospital setting. For example, girls admitted because they were thought to be 'in moral danger' may be given little opportunity as inpatients to hazard their virtue, and patients admitted because they were aggressive towards members of their family may not have the same motives for aggression in the hospital environment. McKerracher, *et al.* (1966) have shown a low prevalence of behaviour disorders amongst patients in Rampton, all of whom would have been admitted initially because of their behaviour.

There was little difference between the sexes in the proportion of disturbed patients, but rather more disorders were reported amongst women and only withdrawal was more frequent amongst males. This is worth remarking, because in the general population aggression and destructive behaviour is commoner amongst males. McKerracher and his colleagues found the same pattern at Rampton and suggested that violent behaviour in male patients, in contrast to that of females, was more commonly a means to a material end, and when benefits were not likely to result it did not occur. Possibly the effect of institutionalization is generally more disturbing to women than it is to men.

Difficult behaviour was related to grade and occurred rather more frequently amongst younger patients than in those over 25 (Table 4.8), and this was due to a fall in its occurrence amongst feeble-minded patients and female imbeciles in the older group. It was most common amongst patients aged 15–25, the group most likely to be admitted for this reason (Leeson, 1963).

We cannot, of course, say from this study how much of the behaviour disorder reported is due to deprivation of affection or lack of occupation or other environmental effects, and how much to causes such as neurological damage. Some researches, however, have shown that institutional living does tend to produce higher rates of disturbed behaviour among the mentally handicapped (Kaufman, 1967), and Tizard (1964) has shown that the behaviour of children transferred from a hospital ward to a small living unit improved. The extent to which the prevalence of disturbance can be reduced by changing patients' social environment will be shown for younger patients by the Wessex experiment (Kushlick, 1969). Our figures show merely what hospitals have to cope with at the present time and provide a base-line for measuring improvements.

PATIENTS' ABILITIES

Impeded as they are by their mental, physical and behavioural handicaps, what can patients in hospital actually do in terms of achieving independence? In the following analysis a patient is rated as completely dependent if he is quite unable to attend to any of his basic needs, i.e. cannot walk even with aid, is incontinent, and cannot feed or dress himself. He is classed as independent if he can walk as least with aid, has bladder and bowel control and can feed and dress himself. Over 60 per cent are independent in these terms, while 36 per cent of patients are incapable of attending to their basic needs in one or more ways, and consequently require some help from nursing staff. Only 5 per cent are totally dependent. Grade is of crucial importance here, for while 29 per cent of idiots are totally dependent and none are independent, 87 per cent of the feeble-minded and 60 per cent of imbeciles are fully independent.

Table 4.10 shows the distribution of dependency by age and grade. In the younger age groups, that is patients aged under 25 years, the percentage of patients who are independent drops to about 36 per cent, while over 12 per cent are completely dependent. This means that in a forty-four-bedded ward (the average ward size for the under 25s), four or five patients will require total care and attention, twenty-four or twenty-five will require some assistance, and only fourteen or fifteen patients will be able to attend to most of their own needs. This obviously represents a very heavy burden on the nursing staff.[5]

There are likely to be three groups of patients who have difficulty in acquiring these basic skills, apart from those few very young children who are not yet sufficiently mature to learn. First, the low-grade patients who are too retarded even to learn simple tasks; these frequently suffer from physical handicaps also. Secondly, patients who have sufficient intellectual ability, but who have some motor or sensory handicap

[5] This illustration is theoretical since in fact wards in subnormality hospitals are not usually arranged in this way, but tend to specialize according to ability, so that all the dependent patients are in wards together.

TABLE 4.10

PERCENTAGE OF PATIENTS IN EACH OF THE GRADE AND AGE GROUPS
COMPLETELY DEPENDENT OR FULLY INDEPENDENT IN BASIC SKILLS

Age in years	0–15	16–25	26–65	66+	Total
Idiots total	41	47	37	1	126
% Completely dependent	39	34	11	—	29
% Independent	0	0	0	—	0
Imbeciles total	75	119	348	41	583
% Completely dependent	7	2	2	2	3
% Independent	23	58	69	76	61
Feeble-minded total	4	58	267	42	371
% Completely dependent	0	0	0	2	1
% Independent	50	86	89	83	87
Total residents	120	224	652	84	1,080
% Completely dependent	17	8	2	4	5
% Independent	16	53	73	79	64

which makes it difficult for them to manipulate objects, especially in view of their limited intelligence. Thirdly, patients who have the ability to learn but who cannot do so with the amount of attention and training which they are given at present, particularly if they are emotionally disturbed. It may not be possible to do much in the way of independence training with the first group, i.e. the very low-grade, especially those with physical handicaps. With a different approach to training, however, it should be possible to overcome the problems of the two latter groups.

The remaining portion of this section will deal with each basic skill in turn and make some assessment of the extent to which those who are at present dependent might be trainable. This is obviously somewhat speculative, because it is impossible to be sure that an individual has the capacity to learn some task until he has proved it by actually doing so. But where the data suggest that many high- and medium-grade patients have not achieved independence, although they are not physically handicapped, one is entitled, perhaps, to wonder whether this state of affairs could be improved.

Eating
Thirteen per cent of residents cannot feed themselves with a spoon, and most of these are of low grade. Table 4.11 shows the relationship between grade and ability to feed oneself, and also gives the percentage of patients in each grade who were unable to feed themselves and suffered from a relevant motor or sensory handicap, i.e. were either blind or had crippled hands. Five of the seven high-grade patients unable to feed

TABLE 4.11

PERCENTAGE OF PATIENTS IN EACH GRADE AND AGE GROUP UNABLE
TO FEED THEMSELVES AND WITH A RELEVANT PHYSICAL HANDICAP

Age in years	0–15	16–25	25+	Total	%
Total idiots	41	47	38	126	100
% Cannot feed self	76	66	63	86	68
% Cannot feed self with relevant handicap	46	36	18	43	34
Total imbeciles	75	119	389	583	100
% Cannot feed self	19	12	6	52	9
% Cannot feed self with relevant handicap	5	5	4	26	4
Total feeble-minded	4	58	309	371	100
% Cannot feed self	0	2	2	7	2
% Cannot feed self with relevant handicap	0	0	2	5	1
Total residents	120	224	736	1,080	100
% Cannot feed self	37	20	7	145	13
% Cannot feed self with relevant handicap	19	10	4	74	7

themselves were physically handicapped, while about half of the idiot and imbecile patients were physically handicapped.

Over 10 per cent of medium-grade patients could not feed themselves. Since feeding with a spoon is a skill acquired by a normal child with a mental age of eighteen months to two years, one would not expect to find such a high proportion of imbecile patients to be incapable of this task. Over half of these patients had a physical handicap which would restrict their ability to learn, although it is possible that even some of these patients could be helped to independence if they received intensive training and were given the special mechanical aids which have been developed for handicapped children of normal intelligence, for example, the swivel spoons developed for limbless 'thalidomide' children. We are not suggesting necessarily that much more could be done to train these patients with the present level of staffing or facilities, but rather that these figures show that only limited results can be achieved given the conditions present in most hospitals.

Dressing

About one-third of patients need help with dressing. Table 4.12 shows the relationship between grade and ability to dress and the percentage of those unable to dress themselves who also suffer from a relevant motor or sensory handicap, i.e. those who are blind or have crippled hands. Dressing oneself, as defined in this survey, i.e. independence except for managing buttons and laces, requires a mental age of about five years and so will be beyond the capacity of some imbeciles, especially those under the age of ten years, and of all idiots, although those without physical handicap may learn at least to co-operate with dressing routines. Most imbecile and feeble-minded patients with a physical handicap may also be unable to acquire this skill, although with special instruction and mechanical aids it may be possible to develop a degree of independence.

Altogether perhaps about one-third of those patients not at present dressing themselves appear to be of imbecile level or above and are without a physical handicap, and one cannot easily account for their failure to acquire this skill. A further 20 per cent probably have sufficient intelligence but have a

TABLE 4.12

PERCENTAGE OF RESIDENTS IN EACH GRADE AND AGE GROUP UNABLE
TO DRESS THEMSELVES AND WITH A RELEVANT PHYSICAL HANDICAP

Age in years	0–15	16–25	25+	Total	%
Idiots total	41	47	38	126	100
% Cannot dress self	100	100	100	126	100
% Cannot dress self with relevant handicap	46	45	32	52	41
Imbecile total	75	119	389	583	100
% Cannot dress self	72	39	24	193	33
% Cannot dress self with relevant handicap	16	13	9	64	11
Feeble-minded total	4	58	309	371	100
% Cannot dress self	25	5	5	21	6
% Cannot dress self with relevant handicap	25	2	3	11	3
Total residents	120	224	736	1,080	100
% Cannot dress self	80	43	20	340	31
% Cannot dress self with relevant handicap	27	16	8	127	12

physical handicap which may limit their capacity to acquire
this skill. Again the figures suggest that not all patients at
present have the opportunity to develop their potential for
independence.

Incontinence

Table 4.13 shows the numbers of incontinent patients in each
mental grade. Almost all idiots are at least singly incontinent
and about three-quarters are doubly incontinent. Among imbeciles and the feeble-minded in particular there is surprisingly
little difference between the numbers doubly and singly incontinent, although in normal development one expects bowel
regulation to precede bladder control. Again the number of
patients who are still dependent right into adolescence, and
who are not physically handicapped, suggests that they may
not have had the opportunity to acquire this skill.

TABLE 4.13

PERCENTAGE OF INCONTINENT PATIENTS IN EACH GRADE AND AGE
GROUP WITH A RELEVANT PHYSICAL HANDICAP

Age in years	0–15	16–25	25+	Total	%
Total idiots	41	47	38	126	100
% Incontinent	100	81	84	111	88
% Incontinent with relevant motor handicap	58	53	42	65	52
Total imbeciles	75	119	389	583	100
% Incontinent	64	23	16	138	24
% Incontinent with relevant motor handicap	20	12	7	56	10
Total feeble-minded	4	58	309	371	100
% Incontinent	25	7	5	21	6
% Incontinent with relevant motor handicap	—	3	3	11	3
Total residents	120	224	736	1,080	100
% Incontinent	75	31	15	270	25
% Incontinent with relevant motor handicap	32	18	7	132	12

TABLE 4.14

PERCENTAGES OF RESIDENTS WHO CAN SPEAK IN SENTENCES, BY
GRADE AND AGE GROUP

Age in years	0–5	6–15	16–25	26–65	66+	Total	%
Imbeciles total	2	73	119	348	41	583	100
% With speech	0	47	65	79	80	419	72
Feeble-minded total	0	4	58	267	42	371	100
% With speech	0	100	100	96	95	359	97
Total population	5	115	224	652	84	1,080	100
% With speech	0	33	61	81	87	773	73

Speech and literacy

Speaking in this survey is defined as the ability to talk in short sentences. This requires a mental age of 2 to $2\frac{1}{2}$ years and so is outside the capacity of idiots.[6]

Table 4.14 shows ability to speak, in relation to age and grade. Nearly three-quarters of all inpatients (and 82 per cent of non-idiots) can speak by this definition. A greater number than this, of course, will be able to comprehend speech or use single words to make their wants known. By far the majority of patients, therefore, are capable of communicating at a simple level and should be capable of benefiting from education and training.

All subjects classified as feeble-minded and under the age of 25 are able to speak, but a smaller number (about 4 per cent) over this age could not do so, presumably as a result of deafness or mental illness. In the imbecile grade, 42 per cent of those under 25 cannot speak in sentences compared with 21 per cent of those over 25 years. But up to the age of 20 the ability to speak increases with each successive five-year age group. There is therefore no reason to suppose that the older patients are of a different kind from those who are younger, but only that they have learned more.

One-quarter of the patients are reported as able to read with fluency (that is simple newspapers and magazines), although this may be unreliable since ward staff may not always know if a patient can read. This is of course quite a high-level skill requiring a mental age of at least 8–9 years. There will be, in addition, a number of patients who can recognize their own names and read words and phrases sufficiently well to cope with life outside a hospital environment. Nurses report that nearly one-third of patients (32·2 per cent) are able to tell the time to within a quarter of an hour, a skill probably indicating a mental age of at least five years.

OCCUPATION

In the preceding sections we examined the extent of handicap in the hospital population, and the proportions of patients who

---

[6] All those subjects classified as idiot by the ward staff, but who could speak in sentences were reclassified as imbecile for the purpose of all analyses. There were, however, only seventeen patients who were reclassified as imbecile for this reason.

at the time of the survey were unable to look after themselves in fundamental ways. In this section we shall look at the proportion of patients who were employed in some way and relate this to handicap in an attempt to assess the adequacy of occupation in quantitative terms.

In the enquiry described in Chapter 3 we were unable to cover every kind of occupation, but it appeared that in the country as a whole about one third of higher-grade patients (i.e. imbeciles and feeble-minded residents) under 16 years of age were not receiving training or education, and that 57 per cent of higher grade adults were without occupation of any kind.

In the ward study we asked staff to report the duration of occupation or education each patient received. No attempt was made in the questionnaire to distinguish between formal industrial or occupational therapy and work in hospital departments or on wards. This was primarily because it is not always possible to distinguish in practice between the two, and a patient may engage in either type of activity, depending on what is available on a particular day. In addition, however, it became apparent at the pilot stage of the enquiry that ward staff did not always know exactly how a patient was occupied when he was off the ward. The pilot study indicated that nurses could reliably report which patients were in school or working outside the hospital, but apart from this we merely asked which patients were occupied in any way within the hospital grounds, for four hours or more each day,[7] for two to four hours, or for less than two hours.

Since no distinction was made between work on the wards, work in a training shop or industrial unit, every type of activity should have been recorded here. Table 4.15 shows the number of patients engaged in any activity, and suggests that 35 per cent of patients are not occupied at all, while a further 11 per cent are occupied for less than four hours a day. Altogether therefore nearly half the population (46 per cent) are either unoccupied or occupied for only a few hours each day.

No idiots were reported to be receiving training or occupa-

[7] Four hours was chosen because it seemed likely, from the way that most hospital mealtimes are arranged, that a four-hour day would involve the patient in some work both morning and afternoon.

TABLE 4.15

NUMBERS AND PERCENTAGES OF PATIENTS BY THE AMOUNT OF
OCCUPATION THEY RECEIVE

Total population		*Total* 1,080	% 100
In school	74*		
Working outside hospital	26	} 595	55
Occupied 4+ hours a day	495		
Occupied 2–4 hours a day	48	} 118	
Occupied 2 hours a day	70		11
Total occupied	713		65
Total unoccupied	382		35

* 15 patients in school were also engaged in some other occupation, but are only included once in this table.

TABLE 4.16

PERCENTAGE OF PATIENTS OCCUPIED BY GRADE

	N	%	*Adequately occupied* %	*Occupied in someway* %	*Unoccupied* %
Idiot	126	100	0	0	100
Imbecile	583	100	52	64	36
Feeble-minded	371	100	77	89	11
Total	1,080	100	55	65	35

tion, and about one-third of all patients not occupied at all are of idiot grade. It may be argued that these patients are too dull to be occupied in any way. Under present hospital conditions this is no doubt true, although the fact that over 30 per cent of them have learnt to feed themselves with a spoon indicates that many are capable of acquiring some simple skills. However, for the most part in this section we shall accept the conventional assumption that idiots are untrainable and therefore exclude them from most of the following analyses. There still remains the problem of why nearly 40 per cent of imbecile and feeble-minded residents between the ages of 5 and 65 are spending all or most of the day without work or education (see Table 4.17).

In the following analyses it is assumed that any imbecile or feeble-minded patient aged 5 years or more, who is under retiring age (65 years), is capable of some occupation, although it may be difficult to employ patients with a motor or sensory handicap. This is not to imply that young children, the old and the handicapped can legitimately be left unoccupied, but simply that there are special problems with these groups and so they must be considered separately. Those patients who are in school, or at work outside the hospital or occupied within the hospital for four hours or more each day, are described as being 'adequately occupied'. Many of these, of course, are not being seriously educated or employed in the sense of being in a school or workshop which employs well-trained and enthusiastic staff, and where there is really an industrious atmosphere. In many of the hospital training departments we visited there was little evidence of the busy, happy environment found in the best Local Authority training centres. There was often an air of despondency, with work proceeding at a desultory pace and some patients actually falling off to sleep from time to time. Furthermore, a twenty-hour week is a very low standard to accept as the minimum for 'adequate' occupation.

TABLE 4.17

PERCENTAGE OF HIGHER-GRADE PATIENTS WHO ARE IN SCHOOL OR 'ADEQUATELY OCCUPIED', BY AGE GROUPS

Ages in years	6–16		17–25		26–65		65+		Total	%
	N	%	N	%	N	%	N	%		
Feeble-minded & imbecile total	104		152		615		83		954	100
In school	57		17		—	—	—	—	74	
'Adequately occupied'	13		76		401		36		526	
Total	70	67	93	61	401	65	36	43	600	63

Bearing these qualifications in mind, however, Table 4.17 presents the number of middle- and high-grade patients between the ages of 5 and 65 who in these terms can be classed as being 'adequately occupied'. Only about 60 per cent of patients in these grades can be termed such, and nearly half of the imbecile patients and about 20 per cent of the feeble-minded within this age range are reported to be inadequately occupied (see Table 4.16). This result was examined further to determine what percentage of inadequately occupied patients suffer from a sensory or motor handicap. Table 4.18 shows that only about one-quarter of the inadequately occupied imbeciles and a third of the feeble-minded were handicapped in any way. It may be that some of the remaining patients are encopretic or subject to very frequent epileptic fits or have severe behaviour disorders. However, these obstacles are not adequate grounds for denying patients occupation, particularly since 60 per cent of the non-handicapped imbecile patients and 86 per cent of the feeble-minded can speak and are therefore clearly within the trainable category.[8] Dr Kushlick's study in Wessex confirms these general findings, since he found only one-third of adult patients in formal training or education, but over 55 per cent of residents were completely independent and without behaviour disorder.

TABLE 4.18

ANALYSIS OF HIGHER-GRADE PATIENTS NOT 'ADEQUATELY OCCUPIED' BY AGE, GRADE AND HANDICAP

Ages in years	Imbeciles 6–65 yrs	Feeble-minded 6–65 yrs	Total 6–65 yrs
Total not 'adequately occupied'	249	66	315
% Sensory or motor handicap	27	30	28
% No sensory or motor handicap and can speak	73	70	72

Considering only the population under 25 years of age, those who are most in need of education and training, over 40 per cent of patients considered eligible were not adequately occupied and over half were not in school. Of feeble-minded and imbecile children aged between 6 and 16 years about 40 per cent were not in school. Even allowing for the high rate of physical handicap in the under-25s, which might make education difficult to organize, these figures suggest a very serious lack of facilities for the education and training of young patients. There were considerable variations between Regions

[8] In fact one-third of all patients who can speak in sentences are not adequately occupied.

in the percentage of patients being educated, although the numbers involved in some cases are small. For example in one Region only half of the high- and medium-grade young patients were adequately occupied, compared with two-thirds in another Region.

Further evidence that the present hospital population is under-occupied comes from examining the situation in one hospital which took part in the survey (Hospital 25) which had excellent school and workshop facilities. The management in this hospital claimed that it was able to occupy in some way every patient who could feed himself with a spoon. The questionnaires returned by Hospital 25 showed this to be true. Whereas in the total hospital population 37 per cent of imbeciles and 11 per cent of feeble-minded patients have no occupation, less than 10 per cent of all patients in Hospital 25 were unoccupied.

This hospital does not have many idiot patients and it has no facilities for very severely handicapped patients. However, even if analysis is limited to residents who can feed themselves and use their hands and who are not blind, in the general hospital population 23 per cent of imbeciles and 12 per cent of feeble-minded patients are totally unoccupied, while *all* patients in this category in Hospital 25 are occupied. All patients in Hospital 25 who can speak are 'adequately occupied', whereas in the general hospital population only 68 per cent of those who can speak are 'adequately occupied'.

This particular hospital is only small (the total number of patients is only 215), and therefore the figures quoted may be subject to some margin of error. It seems likely, however, that this unit is providing occupation and training facilities for patients who in other hospitals would be unemployed. Hospital 25 is justifiably proud of its record (not only in occupying patients but in other respects also), but the questionnaires returned were completed by several different members of staff, and there is no reason to suspect that the facts were misrepresented in any way. Furthermore we visited the school and workshop departments in Hospital 25, as we did in most hospitals, and were greatly impressed not only by the extent of work available but also by quality of work achieved and by the general atmosphere of industry and purposefulness.

STAFFING

Figures showing professional staff by Region for 1969 are quoted in a new Department of Health and Social Security publication (Statistical Report Series No. 10, 1970). These are shown in Table 4.19, quoted as ratios per 100 resident patients.

TABLE 4.19

VARIATIONS BETWEEN THE THREE REGIONS IN THE PROPORTION OF PROFESSIONAL STAFF AVAILABLE

	RHB1	RHB2	RHB3
Consultants*[1]	0·49	0·22	0·17
Qualified nurses[1]	16·30	13·35	13·75
Psychologists[1]	0·01	0·03	0·20
Social workers[1]	0·04	0·08	0·07
Industrial instructors and teachers[1]	0·63	1·18	0·89
Ratio of school staff to residents 0–16 years[2]	1 : 36	1 : 11	1 : 16

Notes: * Includes mental illness, mental handicap, child psychiatry and child guidance clinics.

[1] Staff per 100 resident patients. Taken from the Department of Health Statistical Report Series, No. 10, for the year 1969.

[2] Taken from the Department of Health Staffing Returns for the year 1963.

One can immediately see that there are quite wide variations between Regions, particularly in the ratio of training staff provided. Some hospitals in fact employ nurses in adult-training departments, and these would not appear as instructors in the staffing returns, so the actual ratios are probably better than is here indicated, at least for adult patients.

However we were able to obtain from the D.H.S.S. statistical branch, details of school staff for 1963 (the latest year for which figures were collected in such a way that we could incorporate them into our data). These are shown at the bottom of Table 4.19 as a ratio of non-idiot children.

In view of this piece of evidence alone, one wonders again at the figures quoted in the Department's Statistical Report Series on training facilities, where only 3 per cent of children and 5 per cent of adults without formal training are said to be unoccupied due to lack of facilities (see p. 44).

CONCLUSIONS

This survey revealed quite a high level of physical handicap amongst our sample of residents. Thirty-seven per cent of the sample suffered from some motor or sensory handicap and the proportion was even higher among younger patients (Table 4.5). If patients are to achieve maximum independence, it is necessary to identify those handicaps which are remedial and those which can be alleviated by mechanical aids. There are few facilities at present available to do this, and the staffing figures given in Table 4.19 show that the number of professional training staff in these hospitals is quite inadequate to deal with a problem of this order. The assessment of the extent and nature of individual handicap is a task requiring a specialized team, prepared to use and develop all the available methods of detection and aids to improvement (Hilliard and Kirman, 1966; Koch, *et al.*, 1965).

At the same time it is worth recalling that 64 per cent of residents in our sample are quite independent in being able to look after their basic needs, that over 80 per cent of non-idiot patients can speak in sentences, while nearly 35 per cent of all patients are described as being of at least feeble-minded grade. This suggests that the majority of patients are trainable, and that many should be able to achieve quite a high level of skill, given the proper conditions for learning.

There is evidence here to suggest that at present the opportunity for patients to develop their potential for independence cannot be provided by most hospitals. About one-third of the patients in the sample were unable to attend to one or more of their basic needs, and this represents a very heavy burden on the nursing staff; but a further analysis of the patients unable to care for themselves suggests that the numbers who require help could be reduced. In a survey of this kind estimates of the proportion of patients who are trainable cannot be given with absolute confidence. The identification of individual patients who can be trained is a task for the medical, nursing and educational teams concerned with them. However, if the number of dependent and semi-independent patients can be reduced, the nursing staff will be freed of some of their more onerous and less rewarding duties, and can at the same time concentrate on activities which are more rewarding. Such a change of emphasis would not be easy initially. It often appears less troublesome at the time to feed a young child, or change him, than to make the effort to encourage him to feed himself or use a toilet. With mentally handicapped patients even more effort is required to teach them to be independent, but in the long run this would be beneficial to patients and staff alike.

There are very few studies in this country which quote attempts to develop greater independence among subnormal inpatients by special teaching methods. The Brooklands experiment suggested that this more homely kind of residential unit did allow patients to improve in social behaviour and to become more independent. Furthermore, a study by Lyle comparing children living in their own homes with children in hospital matched on non-verbal I.Q. showed that the children with the advantage of a home environment were more advanced in self-care than the hospital children (Lyle, 1959), and the same pattern is suggested in Tizard and Grad (1961).

Work now coming from the United States, where Skinnerian teaching methods are being applied to the training of the mentally handicapped, is more directly relevant. In these studies psychologists lead programmes for developing various skills in the children, but nurses also are taught how to participate. Very dramatic improvement is reported, even with patients initially testing at I.Q.s well below 40. It could be argued that most of the patients in these American studies were originally living in much worse conditions than are present in the average British hospital, and consequently respond more readily to a retraining programme of any type. However, these studies do suggest ways by which a different approach to training can be initiated, and methods devised which would involve the nursing staff and therefore not require large numbers of specially qualified personnel (McKay and Sidman, 1967; Sidman and Stoddard, 1966; Ullman and Krasner, 1965; Krasner and Ullman, 1965).

Even more indicative perhaps of the inadequate facilities at present provided in hospitals is the data concerning occupation and training. About one-third of all patients who should be eligible for work in terms of their grade and age are not adequately occupied, and many appear to have no occupation at all. Nearly half of those aged between 5 and 16 years are not in school, and very little schooling is available at all for patients over 16 years, although this may well be the age when such patients could benefit most from formal teaching. Again, in an extensive study such as this, one cannot accurately assess the training needs of patients and to what extent these are being fulfilled. But there is surely cause for great concern over the numbers of young patients who are not being taught and are therefore unlikely to have the opportunity to achieve their full potential. With older patients, the situation is more complex. It was shown earlier in the present chapter that over one-half of the medium-grade, and two-thirds of the high-grade patients had been in hospital for over ten years. These are unlikely ever to achieve a fully independent existence, and there is little point in directing their training towards this end. It may be most economical to employ them on contract work in a work-like environment, and patients may be happiest occupied in this way. Alternatively, either or both objectives may be best served by employing them in maintenance and service work about the hospital. It is not obvious which type of employment is more satisfactory to the patient, although in either case incentives are likely to be important (Clarke, 1965). It can hardly be questioned, however, that under-employment will be harmful to the patient, and will produce further deterioration in his condition, although this has been clearly demonstrated only for the mentally ill (Brown and Wing, 1967). A high proportion of patients in our sample were considered to have behaviour disorders, and the most common of these was withdrawal and aggression. It would be a difficult task to demonstrate the extent to which these behaviour patterns are the result of boredom or under-stimulation, but quite dramatic changes have been observed among mentally ill patients in these very characteristics when more stimulation and opportunity for independence was introduced into their wards.

It must be recognized that a substantial proportion of hospital residents, the very low-grade or idiot patients, will never achieve much in the way of independence, and that their main needs will be for total nursing care. It is also probably unrealistic to expect that many medium-grade patients will ever attain full independence, and, even given the maximum amount of training and help, the majority will only function successfully in a sheltered hospital or hostel environment. However, if the aim of a hospital is to develop fully the potential of all their residents and to help them to attain whatever degree of independence they can manage, then the results of our survey suggest that this aim is not being achieved at the present time.

Over 30 per cent of the residents in our sample are of medium and high grade and are under 25 years of age, and therefore should be receiving active training and education at the time when this will be most beneficial. A further 50 per cent of residents are of medium or high grade between age 25 and 65 and should be occupied in some fairly intensive way. One realizes that the existing resources allocated to subnormality hospitals do not allow for this ideal to be achieved, but this must surely, in the long run, be uneconomic as well as inhumane.

Finally, we must consider the needs of the feeble-minded patients who represent about one-third of all residents. It is surprising to find that only a very small proportion of these patients are said to be physically handicapped (28 per cent) or suffering from a behaviour disorder (37 per cent), while the vast majority (87 per cent) are completely independent in their basic needs. One wonders why these patients are considered to be in need of residential care at all, at least within a hospital environment. A more detailed study would be required to decide what alternative arrangements for their care, if any, could be made. But it seems on the face of it unjustifiable on the one hand to have able-bodied adults of reasonable intellectual ability housed within an institution, or on the other hand to have scarce hospital resources devoted to adult 'patients' who seem to be without any obvious need of a hospital bed.

5

A COHORT STUDY OF HOSPITAL FIRST ADMISSIONS

There are a number of basic questions concerning the role of hospitals for the mentally handicapped, which cannot be answered from the evidence of formal hospital statistics or from the results of *ad hoc*, cross-sectional surveys of hospital residents. If we wish to know how many patients remain in hospital at varying intervals after an initial admission, and how likely they are to be re-admitted after discharge, how these contingencies vary according to the patient's mental grade and age at the time of first admission, and, particularly, if we are concerned about the ways in which these patterns of hospital stay may have been modified by changes in treatment and discharge policies – then we must embark on a 'cohort' study. This involves selecting a number of different years, identifying every patient admitted to hospital in a particular area during each of these years, and summarizing the subsequent experience of each of these groups (or cohorts) of patients; it then becomes possible to ascertain how far a patient's chances of being discharged from or remaining within hospital varied according to the year in which he was admitted.

Three years were chosen for the study: 1949, the first calendar year after the inauguration of the National Health Service; 1959, which as well as being a conventional decade later was the last year before the implementation of the Mental Health Act; and 1963, which though closer in time to the middle year of the study than might have been ideal, was the latest year it was possible to study while still leaving adequate time for follow-up. The study was limited to a single but important Region, that of the North-West Metropolitan Hospital Board. This had been one of the three Hospital Regions covered in our review of hospital ward patients, and was one of the largest in the country. It covered a population of more than four millions, and comprised (before the reorganization of London local government in 1965) the Metropolitan Boroughs in the north-west quadrant of the London County Council's area, about four-fifths of Middlesex and large parts of Hertfordshire and Bedfordshire, as well as small sections of the counties of Surrey, Berkshire and Buckinghamshire. About half of the population lived in Middlesex, the area dealt with in the community cohort study in the following chapter.

It is not possible to compare the Region's population with others for any characteristcs, since no relevant figures are published. The fact that it is metropolitan and that half of the catchment area population lives in Middlesex, which as we shall show later was atypical in the community services it provided, must limit to some extent the generalizations which can be made from the study of this Region. However, as we showed in Chapter 3, there appear to be no great differences between Regions in the composition of the hospitalized mentally handicapped, and furthermore the trends in numbers of admissions for the North-West Metropolitan Region are similar to those shown in national statistics.

Details of how this study was organized are contained in Appendix 1. Briefly we identified all patients entering hospitals for the mentally handicapped for the first time in the years specified. We then extracted from their medical records details of the patients' characteristics, length of stay in hospital and their subsequent experience of hospital care throughout the follow-up period, that is from the date of admission until the end of 1965.

CHARACTERISTICS OF THREE ADMISSION
COHORTS

Short-stay and long-term care
It can be seen from Table 5.1 that there was a large overall increase in the number of admissions between 1949 and the two later cohorts. The total number of admissions in 1963 was about 70 per cent greater than in 1949. However, the number of cases admitted for long-term care dropped over the period studied, and it was only the growth in admissions for short-

term care which produced this rise in the total numbers entering hospital.

TABLE 5.1

TOTAL NUMBER OF LONG-TERM AND SHORT-STAY ADMISSIONS FOR EACH COHORT

	1949	1959	1963
Long term	217	203	153
Short term	—	175	200
Total	217	378	353

In Chapter 2, we described the introduction during the early 1950s of informal short-term admission procedures. In 1949 all mentally handicapped patients were admitted and discharged, formally, by legal order. It was therefore difficult to admit patients for a short period only, except for a few hospitals which operated their own informal admission procedures in defiance of the Act. From 1952 when informal admission was officially permitted for short-term care, i.e. for periods of up to eight weeks, the use of this facility developed rapidly. Our cohort study clearly shows this, for by 1959 nearly half of all admissions in the Region studied were short-term cases, and the proportion had increased again by 1963.

Because the formal distinction between long- and short-term care was eliminated by the 1959 Act, it was not always possible in our study of the case notes to distinguish those patients who were admitted with the intention of their remaining in hospital for less than eight weeks from those who, although not admitted on this basis, in fact remained in hospital for a short time only. We have therefore defined as a short-stay patient anyone admitted in 1959 or 1963 whose admission lasted for less than three months. The majority of patients classified as short-stay on this basis were admitted explicitly for short-term care, but some of the high-grade patients in this category may be self-discharges or patients who proved capable of being discharged within three months, although admitted initially for an indefinite period. We did not consider any 1949 patients as 'short-stay' even if they were discharged within three months, but since the number of such patients was very small (less than 8 per cent) this is unlikely to affect the picture to any great extent.

This finding concerning the great increase in the percentage of short-term admissions was the most striking result in our study, and therefore we shall discuss this point fully before going on to discuss grade and age characteristics of admissions. The obvious question to be answered is : how does this type of provision operate, and what kind of patients are using the facility? There are two possibilities :

(a) that it is catering for some types of patient who formerly did not make use of the hospital service. In this case one would expect to find that the number of long-term admissions had remained the same or increased over the period studied, with short-stay admissions additional to this for some specific groups.

(b) that its main function has been to help families to cope with patients formerly admitted for permanent care, but who can be kept at home with increased community provision. This might be indicated where, for certain categories of patient, long-term admissions have declined but short-term admissions have increased.

Looking first at high-grade patients, comparison between the three cohorts shows that for all age groups, except the under fives, there was an increase in both long-term and short-stay admissions (see Table 5.2). For the group aged 16–20 years, there was an increase in long-term admissions and, in addition, there were some short-term admissions. For adult patients, that is those 16 years and over, there was a substantial increase in long-term admissions, with a few short-stay cases also. This would suggest that the overall demand for admission for high-grade patients has increased, especially amongst adults, and that hospital facilities are now being given to patients who would not formerly have been admitted to hospital.

Since there is no reason to suppose that the death rate among high-grade patients has declined dramatically over the years in question, the most likely explanation for this change is a greater willingness to seek admission to hospitals for the mentally handicapped for this grade of patient, when residential care is required. This presumably is partly the result of the easier admission and discharge procedures since the 1959 Act, and partly of the improved environment in many psychiatric hospitals since they came under the National Health Service Act, which have combined to make families and social agencies less fearful of the consequences of admission. Probably the

TABLE 5.2

ANALYSIS OF LONG-TERM AND SHORT-TERM ADMISSIONS BY GRADE AND AGE GROUPS

Age groups	0-5	6-10	11-15	16-20	21-25	26-35	36-45	41-55	56-65	65+
Low and medium-grade admissions 1949	34	35	8	26	3	13	6	6	1	0
Mean long-term admissions 1959-63	20	15	10·5	13·5	3	3·5	4	6	6·5	·5
Mean short-stay admissions 1959-63	52·5	40·5	18·5	3·5	9	5·0	5	3	2·0	·5
(combined)	72	55·5	28	17	12·5	8·5	9	10	7·5	1
High-grade admissions 1949	4	1	3	38	4	3	2	0	0	0
Mean long-term admissions 1959-63	1	2·5	4·5	41·5	8·5	5·5	5·5	5·0	4	1·5
Mean short-term admissions 1959-63	2·5	1·5	2·0	8·5	4·5	3·5	5·0	2·5	1	2·0
(combined)	3·5	3	6·5	50	13	13·5	10·5	7·5	5	3·5

increase in the number of high-grade patients actually resident in hospital is not so great as might appear from looking at admission figures only, as will be shown later. This is because the easier discharge procedures in the later period under study have resulted in shorter stays in hospital for most high-grade patients, with a few being continually re-admitted when formerly they would have been admitted only once on a permanent legal order.

For low- and medium-grade patients slightly different patterns occur for different age groups. Short-stay care was more commonly used for low-grade children than for any other group, and they formed approximately 60 per cent of all short-stay admissions in 1959 and 1963. Indeed for this age group (i.e. low-grade patients under 16 years) there was a drop in the number of long-term admissions over the period studied, but such large numbers of short-stay cases were admitted in 1959 and 1963 that, overall, the number of admissions increased substantially compared with 1949. This suggests that low-grade children, who are difficult to care for at home and who would in the past have been admitted permanently to hospital, can now be managed in the community, presumably because of improved services, although they require periods of temporary inpatient care. However, it remains to be seen whether these patients will ultimately require full-time residential placement as they get older and the problems of home management increase.

For the group aged 16 to 35 years, although the number of total admissions remained substantially the same over the period studied, the number of long-term admissions dropped. By 1959 and 1963 half of the admissions for this age group were short-stay only. If in the future the children admitted for short-term care require long-term care as they grow older, one would expect long-term admissions to rise again for this age group. There is some indication that this is likely to occur from the analysis of re-admissions discussed later on in this chapter.

For low- and medium-grade patients over 35 years, long-term admissions increased slightly over the period studied, and since short-stay cases in 1959 and 1963 were almost as numerous as long-stay cases, this produced an overall increase in admissions for this age group. This probably reflects both the increased life-expectancy of low-grade patients and the increased willingness of families to accept hospital admission, at least on a short-term basis, for their adult low-grade relatives. To this extent short-stay care may be also providing for a type of older patient who formerly never used the hospital service. It also suggests a general increase in the demand for hospital care for this age group.

It would appear therefore that, in the Region studied, short-term care was used primarily for the care of young low-grade patients, for whom long-term admission was much less common in more recent years than in 1949. For low- and medium-grade patients over the age of 35 years and for all high-grade patients, except the under-5s, long-term admission increased over the period under review, and short-stay care was developed supplementary to this. One would expect that, in the future, while short-term admission will remain an important adjunct to community care, especially for low-grade children, long-term admissions will begin to increase again for low-grade patients in the older age groups, when they will probably become too difficult to care for at home.

In view of the importance of short-term admission in the two later cohorts, it would be useful to know in more detail how this facility has affected families at a practical level. Even with the help of community services, the care of low-grade children at home must present considerable difficulties, and the question is whether short-term care was used primarily as a means of relieving pressure on the hospital waiting-list, and thus masking a demand for more permanent beds for these children, rather than to meet the real needs of mentally handicapped patients and their families. Probably the system of short-term care was intended to serve both ends, and so a more important question would be to what extent it has been successful on each count. The description of changes in the demand for hospital care within the county of Middlesex given in the next chapter perhaps throws some light on the possible effect upon families of hospital admission policies.

OTHER CHARACTERISTICS OF ADMISSION

When first admissions for the three cohort years are compared by grade and age on admission, the trends which appear are not large (see Table 5.3). It is the fairly consistent distribution

D

TABLE 5.3

PERCENTAGE OF PATIENTS ADMITTED BY GRADE, SEX AND AGE GROUP

	5 or under M	F	6–10 M	F	11–15 M	F	16–20 M	F	21–25 M	F	25+ M	F	Total
1949													
Low grade	7	2	4	1	—	0·5	0·5	—	—	0·5	0·5	0·5	17
Medium grade	2	3	7	3	2	0·5	5	2	1	0·5	5	5	36
High grade	1	1	0·5	—	1	1	11	6	3	1	8	5	38
Others	1	0·5	0·5	—	1	—	2	1	—	0·5	1	2	9
													100 (N = 217)
1959													
Low grade	3	4	1	1	—	—	—	1	—	—	—	—	10
Medium grade	5	6	7	5	7	2	3	3	1	2	5	5	51
High grade	—	1	1	—	—	1	7	6	2	1	6	7	32
Others	2	1	1	—	—	—	—	2	—	—	1	1	8
													100 (N = 378)
1963													
Low grade	3	3	2	2	—	—	1	2	—	—	—	—	11
Medium grade	4	3	6	4	3	2	4	5	2	1	3	3	36
High grade	1	—	1	—	2	—	9	2	2	2	4	4	30
Others	6	2	2	1	1	—	—	—	—	—	2	3	19
													100 (N = 352)

of age and grade groups within all three cohorts which is of greater interest; in particular the characteristics of the patients admitted in 1959 and 1963 are almost identical, in terms of both numbers and proportions. The most notable difference is the rise over the whole period in the numbers and percentages of admissions of patients under 16 years – 39 per cent in 1949 to 48 per cent in 1959 and 1963 – although of course most of these are short-stay cases.

Surprisingly there is no evidence of a reduction in the admission of patients who were graded as 'normal' in intelligence from the information given in their case-notes. The total numbers involved are of course very small – there were fifteen in 1949, twenty-nine in 1959 and forty-four in 1963. The increase may be, in part, an unreal one, created by the misclassification of patients in 1949, since there was relatively little information in the case notes at that time on which to make a judgement of the patient's abilities, and the resulting tendency may well have been to underestimate the patient's capacities. Some errors in classification are therefore inevitable, but at the same time the I.Q. data where they exist seem to indicate that this impression may be correct. In 1963 only half of all patients had an intelligence test result quoted in their case-notes, and an even greater percentage were apparently untested in the earlier years. However, a check on the number of patients with tested I.Q.s within the normal range in each cohort supported the suggestion that there was no decline in the number of patients of normal intelligence admitted in the later years.

TABLE 5.4

NUMBER OF PATIENTS WITH HIGH I.Q.S ON ADMISSION, IN EACH COHORT

I.Q.	1949	1959	1963
70+	15	29	44
75+	5	18	32
80+	3	2	16

The Region that we studied has two units within large hospitals which specialize in the care of patients who might be classified as 'psychopathic' or 'disturbed'. From the evidence available on reasons for admission, discussed in the next section, there appears to have been a policy in these hospitals of taking high-grade and 'normal' patients who were social misfits, particularly if they were aggressive or broke the law and did not have an adequate home. It does seem likely that, once a hospital acquires a reputation for admitting this kind of person, i.e. the disturbed adolescent or young adult with an inadequate home background, social agencies may opt for admission to such a hospital in cases where the only alternative is prison or Borstal, and this situation no doubt reflects the paucity of residential provision for such cases. The majority of these patients, even those classified here as long-term cases, remain in hospital for a very short time compared with the other grades, and of the 1963 admissions about 60 per cent had been discharged by the end of the follow-up period.

The pattern of admission differs greatly for each grade. About half of the low-grade patients first admitted to hospital were under the age of five years, and nearly 90 per cent under the age of ten. Almost half of the medium-grade patients were first admitted before they were ten years old, and three-quarters before the age of twenty. By contrast, most high-grade patients were over the age of fifteen at first admission and 40 per cent were admitted in a very narrow age group, between the age of 16 and 20 years.

SOURCES OF AND REASONS FOR ADMISSION

We were able to establish the sources of admission for the majority of patients, particularly in the two later cohorts. 'Source of admission' here means the social agency which referred the patient for admission to hospital. In all three cohorts the main source of referral was the Local Authority Mental Health Department, which referred about 60 per cent of long-term and 80 per cent of short-term cases. A further 10 per cent were admitted through the police or courts or from prison or approved school, and this type of admission increased in number over the period studied. This suggests again that hospitals for the mentally handicapped are seen as an alternative to penal care for the socially disturbed young person, especially if he is mentally or educationally backward. A further 5 per cent were admitted from other sources, from hospitals or from general practitioners and occasionally from the Children's Department (see Table 5.5).

The reason why admission was sought was often not stated

TABLE 5.5

SOURCE OF ADMISSION FOR EACH COHORT

		1959		1963	
Source	1949	Long-term	Short-stay	Long-term	Short-stay
Local health authority	125	120	141	92	178
Police	23	23	2	36	7
Approved school/prison	3	0	1	3	1
Other reference	9	9	6	11	8
Not known	57	51	25	11	6
Total	217	203	175	153	200

in the case-notes, particularly in 1949. Even in 1959 and 1963 no reason for admission was given for about 50 per cent of cases. Many of these were of very low grade or with a physical handicap, and this in itself may be taken as a sufficient explanation of admission, but there remain a fairly large number for whom no reason could be elicited from the case-note material; this obviously makes all analyses very unreliable. However it might be worth while stating briefly the main reasons given for admission, relating these to grade and type of admission.

The most common reason given for both high- and low-grade patients is either that the parents were unable to cope, or that the patient's behaviour was difficult. This accounts for nearly half of the reasons given (see Table 5.6). Another common ground for admission, especially among low-grade patients, is some family crisis, e.g. that a mother is ill or confined etc., or the family intention to take a holiday.

There are quite marked differences in the kinds of reasons given for the admission of long-term patients as compared with short-term cases (see Table 5.6). The most common reason given for long-term admission is the inadequacy of the patient's home, where the patient is described as having no home or an inadequate home, or a broken home or where the parents are dead. The second most common reason is that the patient is socially disturbed, aggressive or delinquent or beyond the control of his family. These patients are mainly aged between 10 and 25 years years and are graded imbeciles or feeble-minded. A small number in addition, mostly aged between 16 and 25 years, are said to have been guilty of some breach of the sexual code, rarely an actual offence and usually of a relatively minor kind which one might have supposed capable

TABLE 5.6

REASONS FOR ADMISSION FOR LONG-TERM AND SHORT-STAY CASES, ALL COHORTS COMBINED

	Long-stay	Short-stay
Inadequate home	136	27
Patient's behaviour	130	64
'Parents cannot cope'	68	129
Family crisis	44	30
Other	34	25
Not known	180	81
Total	592	356

of being dealt with quite adequately within the community, if the family were in a position to assume responsibility for the patient's supervision. In quite a large proportion of cases, therefore, it seems that long-term admission was sought primarily because there was no other residential placement available for patients whose own homes were defunct or inadequate, or whose behaviour made it necessary that they be cared for in a more controlled environment. It must be considered whether in these cases a hospital for the mentally handicapped is necessarily the best place to care for these patients. Possibly this is so; but a case could be made for the view that hostel placement for these patients might be more beneficial and more appropriate to their needs.

SUBSEQUENT EXPERIENCE OF HOSPITAL ADMISSIONS

We turn now to consider what happened to patients in each cohort of admissions after they entered hospitals for the mentally handicapped. What proportions remained in hospital, died or were discharged to the community at successive intervals after admission to hospital, and how did these proportions vary according to mental grade and age at admission? In making comparisons between cohorts it should be remembered that differences between cohorts in characteristics were small, and in themselves did not in any way suggest that the need for hospitalization had been reduced to any great extent.

Diagram 5.1 shows the proportion of each cohort in hospital at three-monthly intervals after first admission. This covers all subsequent hospital experience until 1965, and not only the

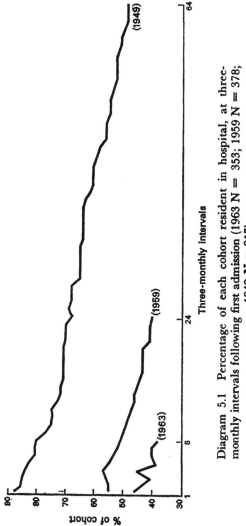

Diagram 5.1 Percentage of each cohort resident in hospital, at three-monthly intervals following first admission (1963 N = 353; 1959 N = 378; 1949 N = 217)

outcome of the initial admission. There was a substantial reduction in the amount of time patients spent in hospital over this period. The evidence is that the proportion of patients admitted who remained in hospital subsequently declined more rapidly in 1959 than in 1949, and still more rapidly in 1963. This is due mainly to discharges of short-term admissions, although some of these patients later returned to hospital again. More importantly, there is also a difference between 1949 and the later cohorts, even if only long-term admissions are considered (see Diagram 5.2), although this effect is much smaller.

The progressive acceleration in the rate at which patients left hospital was due, as might be expected, to an increase in the proportion returning to the community and not to any increase in the death rate of patients in hospital. The only groups of patients who showed a clear difference in the death rate – those admitted before they were five years old and those who were of very low-grade – experienced a declining death rate. In no group did an *increase* in the death rate contribute to the change (see Diagram 5.3).[1]

The decline in the percentage of each cohort resident in hospital at any subsequent point in time occurred in every age group and for each mental grade. However there was little difference between the 1959 and the 1963 cohorts for patients admitted between the ages of 10 and 20 years, and only small differences for low-grade and normal patients.

The experience of the youngest patients – those under five years – and of those aged between 15 and 20 years is shown in detail, both because they include larger numbers of patients than any other five-year group, and because in terms of grade they represent opposite extremes. Thus most of the patients first admitted to hospital before they were five years old were low- or medium-grade, while most of those first admitted between 15 and 20 years were high-grade.

Comparing cohorts, it can be seen that for those admitted first under the age of five years there was a successive decline

[1] The calculations of death rates are based on deaths occurring in hospital plus deaths occurring in the community which were recorded in the case-notes. On the assumption that there was some under-recording of deaths outside hospital, true death rates are presumably somewhat higher than are here shown. Furthermore, since the later cohorts spent less time in hospital, the true death rates for these years are likely to be proportionately higher than those shown, so that the real difference between cohorts may be rather less than is apparent here.

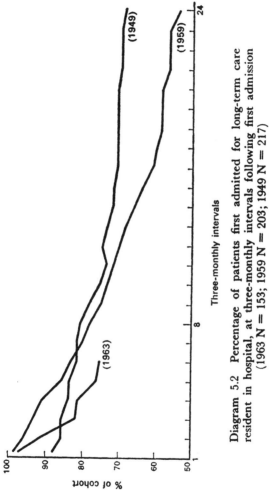

Diagram 5.2 Percentage of patients first admitted for long-term care resident in hospital, at three-monthly intervals following first admission (1963 N = 153; 1959 N = 203; 1949 N = 217)

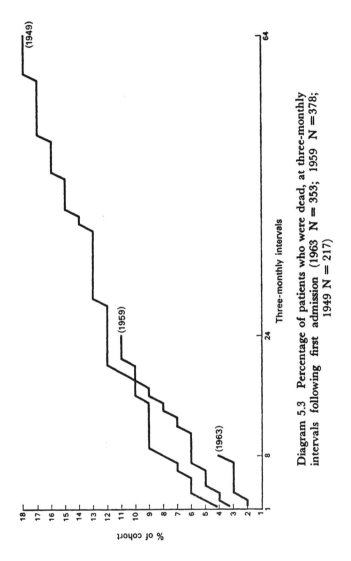

Diagram 5.3 Percentage of patients who were dead, at three-monthly intervals following first admission (1963 N = 353; 1959 N = 378; 1949 N = 217)

between cohort years in the proportions resident in hospital (see Diagram 5.4a). By contrast, for the 15- to 20-year group, there was a marked decline between 1949 and 1959, but thereafter little change in the numbers resident, and the rate of discharge shown for the 1959 and 1963 cohorts is very similar (see Diagram 5.4b).

However, looking at each cohort over time, and considering all patients admitted under the age of 15, there was, in the later cohorts, an initial decline in the percentage of time spent in hospital followed by an increase, especially for patients in the lower grades. This was due to the re-admission of some patients who had been admitted first for short-term care. The proportion of first admissions, for short-term care, in this age group to be found in hospital gradually increased over the follow-up period (see Diagram 5.5). Two years after admission one-quarter of the younger patients first admitted on a temporary basis in 1959 and one-fifth of those admitted in 1963 were resident in hospital. Six years after first admission almost one-third of the 1959 short-stay children were in hospital. This shows that for a substantial proportion of short-stay patients long-term residential care eventually became necessary.

The subsequent experience of the patients admitted during the three key years is summarized in Tables 5.7 and 5.8. These

TABLE 5.7

NUMBERS AND PERCENTAGES OF PATIENTS IN HOSPITAL AT SPECIFIED
PERIODS AFTER FIRST ADMISSION, FOR EACH COHORT

	1949		1959		1963	
	N	%	N	%	N	%
Initial cohort	217	100	378	100	353	100
In hospital at 2 years	176	81	194	51	135	38
Dead at 2 years	17	8	22	6	15	4
Out of hospital	24	11	162	43	203	58
In hospital at 6 years	148	68	151	40	—	—
Dead at 6 years	27	12	43	11	—	—
Out of hospital	42	20	184	49	—	—
In hospital at 16 years	106	49	—	—	—	—
Dead at 16 years	39	18	—	—	—	—
Out of hospital	72	33	—	—	—	—

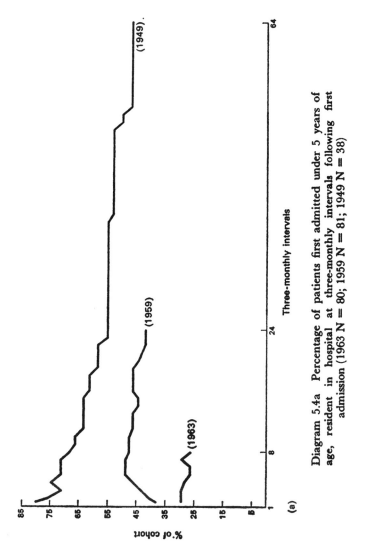

Diagram 5.4a   Percentage of patients first admitted under 5 years of age, resident in hospital at three-monthly intervals following first admission (1963 N = 80; 1959 N = 81; 1949 N = 38)

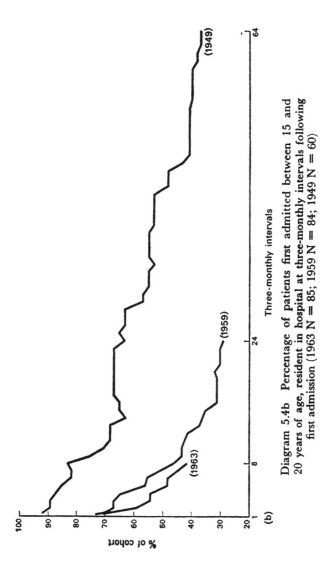

Diagram 5.4b Percentage of patients first admitted between 15 and 20 years of age, resident in hospital at three-monthly intervals following first admission (1963 N = 85; 1959 N = 84; 1949 N = 60)

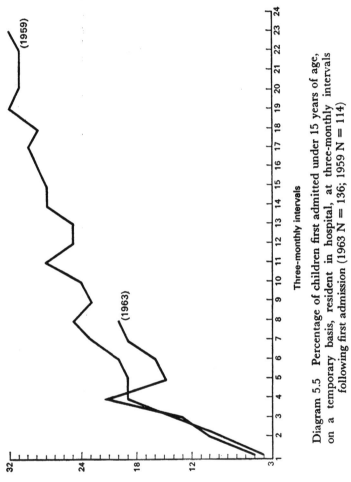

Diagram 5.5   Percentage of children first admitted under 15 years of age, on a temporary basis, resident in hospital, at three-monthly intervals following first admission (1963 N = 136; 1959 N = 114)

TABLE 5.8

NUMBERS AND PERCENTAGES OF PATIENTS IN HOSPITAL AT SPECIFIED
PERIODS AFTER FIRST ADMISSION, FOR EACH COHORT BY AGE GROUP

	1949		1959		1963	
0–5 *years old*	N	%	N	%	N	%
Initial cohort	38	100	81	100	80	100
In hospital at 2 years	26	68	38	47	21	26
Dead at 2 years	10	26	10	12	7	9
Out of hospital	2	6	33	41	52	65
In hospital at 6 years	21	55	34	42	—	—
Dead at 6 years	14	37	16	20	—	—
Out of hospital	3	8	31	38	—	—
In hospital at 16 years	18	47	—	—	—	—
Dead at 16 years	16	42	—	—	—	—
Out of hospital	4	11	—	—	—	—
5–10 *years old*						
Initial cohort	36	100	57	100	65	100
In hospital at 2 years	31	86	25	44	25	38
Dead at 2 years	1	3	2	4	4	6
Out of hospital	4	11	30	52	36	56
In hospital at 6 years	30	83	25	44	—	—
Dead at 6 years	2	6	3	5	—	—
Out of hospital	4	11	29	51	—	—
In hospital at 16 years	21	58	—	—	—	—
Dead at 16 years	7	19	—	—	—	—
Out of hospital	8	23	—	—	—	—
10–15 *years old*						
Initial cohort	12	100	41	100	33	100
In hospital at 2 years	9	75	21	51	16	48
Dead at 2 years	—	—	—	—	1	3
Out of hospital	3	25	20	49	16	49
In hospital at 6 years	8	67	21	51	—	—
Dead at 6 years	—	—	1	2	—	—
Out of hospital	4	33	19	47	—	—

TABLE 5.8—*Continued*

10–15 *years old cont.*	1949 N	%	1959 N	%	1963 N	%
In hospital at 16 years	8	67	—	—	—	—
Dead at 16 years	—	—	—	—	—	—
Out of hospital	4	33	—	—	—	—
15–20 *years old*						
Initial cohort	60	100	84	100	85	100
In hospital at 2 years	50	83	39	46	36	43
Dead at 2 years	1	2	—	—	2	2
Out of hospital	9	15	45	54	47	55
Hospital at 6 years	38	63	24	29	—	—
Dead at 6 years	2	3	—	—	—	—
Out of hospital	20	34	60	71	—	—
In hospital at 16 years	22	37	—	—	—	—
Dead at 16 years	2	3	—	—	—	—
Out of hospital	36	60	—	—	—	—
20 *years old* +						
Initial cohort	71	100	115	100	90	100
In hospital at 2 years	60	84	71	62	37	41
Dead at 2 years	5	7	10	8	1	1
Out of hospital	6	9	34	30	52	58
In hospital at 6 years	51	72	47	41	—	—
Dead at 6 years	9	12	23	20	—	—
Out of hospital	11	15	45	39	—	—
In hospital at 16 years	37	52	—	—	—	—
Dead at 16 years	14	19	—	—	—	—
Out of hospital	20	29	—	—	—	—
35 *years old* +						
Initial cohort	31	100	69	100	45	100
In hospital at 2 years	26	84	48	70	21	47
Dead at 2 years	5	16	10	14	1	2
Out of hospital	—	—	11	16	23	51
In hospital at 6 years	23	71	30	43	—	—
Dead at 6 years	8	26	22	33	—	—
Out of hospital	—	—	17	24	—	—

TABLE 5.8—*Continued*

35 *years old+ cont.*	1949		1959		1963	
	N	%	N	%	N	%
In hospital at 16 years	17	55	—	—	—	—
Dead at 16 years	11	35	—	—	—	—
Out of hospital	3	10	—	—	—	—

show that the *percentage* to be found in hospital following first admission was smaller for the later cohorts than for those admitted in 1949 but, because of the much larger number of patients admitted in the later years, the *absolute numbers* of patients resident in hospital did not fall until after 1963. In particular for most children (except those aged 5 to 10 years) and for patients aged over 35 at admission in 1959, greater numbers resided in hospital six years after admission than was the case for similar patients who were first admitted in 1949. However, comparing the 1963 with the 1949 cohort two years after admission, fewer of the 1963 admissions remained in hospital in all categories, with the exception of children between 10 and 15 years and patients of normal intelligence. This points to a probable future *decline* in the hospital population, unless the lower-grade and youngest patients return to hospital in increasing numbers as they reach adolescence. This latter possibility cannot be estimated from the present data, because none of the youngest patients in the later cohorts was more than 11 years old at the time of follow-up, but it would be wise to interpret any decline in hospital residents with caution until we understand more of the dynamics of the situation.

COMPOSITION OF THE HOSPITAL POPULATION

It is often said by those who work in hospitals that the composition of the hospital population has been changing so as to include an increasing proportion of low-grade patients, and this impression is supported by national figures of patient-flow as well as by the surveys of residents quoted in Chapter 2 and the data presented in Chapter 4. It is also claimed that the children's wards have become 'silted up', because many of those low-grade children who would have died young in earlier years are now surviving at least to adolescence as a result of improved medical care. Table 5.9 shows the number of patients of each grade as a percentage of all patients in hospital two years and six years after admission. Percentages fluctuate somewhat over the three cohorts, but there is no evidence of an increase in low-grade patients as a percentage of residents, whether successive cohorts are compared or the experience of the same cohort is examined over time. In fact there was a fall in their absolute numbers, as already described.

TABLE 5.9

PATIENTS IN EACH GRADE AS A PROPORTION OF ALL PATIENTS
RESIDENT AT SPECIFIED PERIODS AFTER FIRST ADMISSION

	Idiots		Imbeciles		Feeble-minded		Normal		Total	
1949	N	%	N	%	N	%	N	%	N	%
At first admission	36	17	80	37	68	31	14	6	217	100
In hospital at 2 years	26	15	69	39	50	28	14	8	176	100
In hospital at 6 years	22	15	64	43	38	26	9	6	148	100
1959										
At first admission	38	10	191	51	93	25	28	7	378	100
In hospital at 2 years	17	9	95	49	56	29	14	7	194	100
In hospital at 6 years	17	11	84	56	36	24	4	3	151	100
1963										
At first admission	43	12	124	35	68	19	44	12	353	100
In hospital at 2 years	17	13	46	34	25	19	20	15	135	100

N.B. Patients of unspecified grade have been included in the total.

This evidence conflicts with changes shown by surveys of complete hospital populations. Tizard and O'Connor (1964) found 6 per cent of the 1952 population of London hospitals for the mentally handicapped to be idiots, while more recent studies, including that described in Chapter 4, have shown some 12 per cent to be of low grade. In the present enquiry, if only those who were definitely low-grade are considered, the two later cohorts showed around 12 per cent of residents to be low-grade – a reduction on the 1949 figures. But if to this group are added patients whose grade could not be accurately established but who were of low- or medium-grade, then about 20 per cent of residents in the 1949 and 1963 cohorts and around 12 per cent in the 1959 series were of low-grade or idiot level. In either case the considerable changes which led to a general increase in the number of low-grade

TABLE 5.10

PATIENTS IN EACH AGE GROUP ON ADMISSION, AS A PERCENTAGE OF ALL PATIENTS RESIDENT, AT SPECIFIED PERIODS AFTER FIRST ADMISSION

	0–5 years		−10 years		−15 years		−20 years		20+		Total		35 years +	
	N	%	N	%	N	%	N	%	N	%	N	%	N	%
1949														
At first admission	38	17	36	17	12	6	60	28	71	33	217	100	31	14
In hospital at 2 years	26	15	31	18	9	5	50	28	60	34	176	100	26	15
In hospital at 6 years	21	14	30	20	8	5	38	26	51	34	148	100	23	16
1959														
At first admission	81	21	57	15	41	11	84	22	115	30	378	100	69	18
In hospital at 2 years	38	20	25	13	21	11	39	20	71	37	194	100	48	25
In hospital at 6 years	34	23	25	19	21	14	24	16	47	31	151	100	30	20
1963														
At first admission	80	23	65	18	33	9	85	24	90	26	353	100	45	13
In hospital at 2 years	21	16	25	19	16	12	36	27	37	27	135	100	21	16

patients as a percentage of all those in hospital in the 1950s and early 1960s must have occurred in this Region before 1949. The quoted surveys of hospital populations have also shown a decline in the number of high-grade patients in hospital from a level of 50 per cent to 33 per cent of residents. In the present study, however, the proportion remained close to one-third of residents in all three cohorts, although there was evidence of a reduction in the proportion of all residents which they formed following the two-year interval after admission.

Table 5.10 shows the distribution of age groups at admission as proportions of all residents two, six and sixteen years later. Except actually at the point of admission, there is no clear increase in the fraction made up of the youngest patients (those aged under 5 years), either between cohorts, or over time in the same cohort. However, taking all patients under 15 years at first admission, an increase in the percentage of residents formed by this group did occur both between cohorts and over time. It occurs between cohorts because they comprised an increasing proportion of admissions, and it occurs over time because of the reduction in the proportion of residents formed by the 15 to 35-year group.

Patients aged over 35 years of age at admission are of particular interest because of their increasing numbers in national admissions over the period 1959–60. In fact, although in our study they formed a higher proportion of the 1959 residents than of the 1949 residents, by 1963 they made up proportions almost identical to those found in the 1949 series. Again, there is no clear evidence that they increased as a percentage of residents when the same cohort is examined over time.

CONCLUSIONS

The size of the hospital population is the outcome of the number of admissions together with the length of time patients remain in hospital. In the North West Metropolitan Region first admissions increased by 60 per cent between 1949 and the later years, due entirely to the increased use of short-term care. Over the same period, 1949 to 1963, there was an acceleration in the rate at which cohorts of first admissions left hospital, largely for the same reason. On this evidence alone a decline in the resident population should have appeared in the early 1960s; although the effect of these factors might have been offset at first by the large *number* of patients remaining in hospital for the first few years after the peak admission period, in 1959.

By 1965, however, at the end of the follow-up period, none of the youngest and most handicapped of the patients admitted in the later years had reached adolescence, and it is possible that at this age they imposed an increasing burden on their parents and so the pressure for their re-admission increased. By 1967 children who were 5 years old in 1957, when the first special care units were introduced into Middlesex, would have reached the age of 15, and from then on it is likely that low-grade patients returned permanently to hospital in increasing numbers.

How far is this situation reflected at the national level? It is only possible to guess at the answer from the hospital admission and population figures. The peak year for admissions in England and Wales seems to have occurred later than in the Region we studied. There was no marked decline in the hospital population although there was a slight trough in 1965, which may have been the delayed result of an apparent fall in admissions between 1963 and 1964, and of an increase in patient turnover. Thereafter nationally admissions increased, and so, after 1965, did the resident population. It is not possible to say from the figures published whether the increase in admissions was due largely to an increase in adolescent low-grade patients admitted.

The effects of the use of short-term care are the most obvious outcome of this analysis. But a second complementary feature is the slow attrition of the earliest cohort. Sixteen years after admission, 49 per cent of the 1949 patients were still in hospital. The present figures suggest that their numbers will fall, but according to the study described in Chapter 4, patients who have been in hospital for sixteen years or more form one-third of hospital residents. Unless other forms of residential care are developed for older patients therefore the number of patients requiring places in hospital is likely to remain fairly large. It seems evident that most of these patients will not now be able to live outside a sheltered environment, or return to their families, and plans for the care of the mentally handicapped must surely take their situation into account.

6

A COHORT STUDY OF REFERRALS TO
A LOCAL HEALTH AUTHORITY

The proportion of patients admitted to hospital who remain there for any length of time has shown a dramatic decline since 1949, although the numbers of first admissions have increased since then. What changes, if any, in the community might account for these two facts? The evidence from official statistics suggests that it is the increase in community services which has made a speedier turnover possible, and which in turn allows for a greater number of admissions – of which most in recent years have been for periods of up to two months only. However there are other possible explanations which should be considered first, before it can be concluded that it is indeed the expansion of the community services which has produced this change.

To find out what changes have taken place in community care we examined the experience of a sample of primary referrals to the former Middlesex Local Health Authority during the years 1949, 1959 and 1963. Middlesex was chosen as the field of study mainly on practical grounds. But the same choice might have been made for another and theoretically good reason. Middlesex was known, for some years before its disintegration into the nine new London boroughs in 1965, to have a Health Authority which paid particular attention to the care of the mentally handicapped in the area. It was at least one of the first and foremost in developing and extending training and placement facilities in the community. This is illustrated by Diagram 6.1 which shows the growth in the percentage of Middlesex patients receiving training in comparison with the growth in England and Wales as a whole. Although Middlesex figures are not available before 1959, the indications are that this Health Authority had already

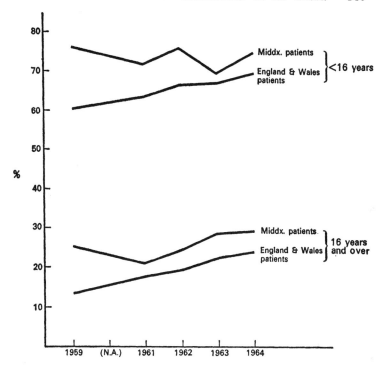

Diagram 6.1 Percentage of Middlesex patients in training-centres compared with the percentage of patients in England and Wales receiving training, between 1959 and 1964

approached, by the second half of the 1950s, what is now the national aim in training provision, at least for patients under 16 years of age. If a high level of provision of community care does affect the demand for hospital care, this should be demonstrable in Middlesex between 1949 and 1963.

Nevertheless the full effects of the new policy would not necessarily be shown during this time period. A patient referred at the age of 5 years in 1959 and admitted early to a training centre would have been only 11 years old at the time of follow-up in 1965, and the effects of early training on his capacity to function as an adult in the community or upon his later need for hospital care would not be known. On the other hand a similar patient referred in 1949 might not have received training until much later in his life, when the number of training-centre places increased. It is, of course, possible to look at the smaller number of 1949 patients who did receive training from an early age, but it is by no means certain that the quality of training was at all comparable in the early 1950s with that which was developed later. Some indication that the function of training-centres in the area was differently conceived, and that therefore a different type of activity was provided before 1955, is given by the fact that until that year they were known as *occupation* centres. However, even given this limitation, it should be possible to find with some certainty whether increased provision of training and other facilities affects the demand for hospital care amongst younger patients.

That Middlesex was atypical in being progressive in the provision of community services is an advantage for the purposes of this study, because it shows the direction in which the findings may be generalized. Atypicality in demographic and epidemiological factors, however, could limit the generalizations which may be made, and it is important that these should be considered.

Middlesex was one of the largest Local Health Authorities in the country, with a population of over two million in 1961. No direct evidence is available on the *incidence* of mental handicap in different areas of the country, but considering the rates per thousand of congenital defects of the central nervous system, which might affect the number of subnormal births, it appears that Middlesex may have a lower incidence of severe mental handicap than elsewhere, because the incidence of these defects in South-East England is relatively low. This suggestion is not out of keeping with the relatively low prevalence rate shown for Middlesex (Tizard and Grad, 1961), although prevalence does not necessarily vary proportionately with incidence. In so far as prevalence determines demand for services at a given point in time, Middlesex might be expected to generate a lower level of demand for services in relation to the total population than other areas. For example, given a population of 200,000 of the relevant age group, and assuming that all the mentally handicapped require training, the Middlesex prevalence rate of 3·45 per 1,000 would generate a demand for 78 places fewer than a rate of 3·84 per 1,000, which is the figure quoted by Kushlick for the Wessex Counties (but for an older age group).

However, when we are discussing patterns of care, the

incidence or prevalence of mental handicap is of less importance than the proportion of any cohort of referrals who require some form of care. Two purely demographic factors affect this proportion, namely death rates and emigration rates. The crude death rate for Middlesex is not much lower than for the whole country, but the emigration rate is higher than for most areas. It follows that, if death or emigration rates for the mentally handicapped parallel those for the general population, the demand for care amongst a cohort of mentally handicapped referrals in Middlesex would decrease more rapidly than in the country generally.[1] For this reason and because of the apparently low prevalence, the *demand* for services in relation to the parent population of the cohorts studied may be lower than would be expected in the country generally. However, there is no reason to assume that the *pattern* of the services and the way in which they appear to interact was unique to Middlesex, although the effects demonstrated would have predated those in most other areas.

In this chapter we compare first the characteristics of the three cohorts of referrals, and secondly the patterns of care which each experienced. The patients studied were drawn from an alphabetical list of patients first referred to the Middlesex Health Authority in 1949, 1959 and 1963 as mentally handicapped, and who had not previously been referred to any other health authority as mentally handicapped. To reduce the numbers in the study to a manageable size, it was necessary to sample, and every second patient aged less than 16 years was included as well as every fourth patient aged 16 years and over. The figures quoted in the text and in tables and diagrams are always weighted to produce approximately the numbers in the original population from which the sample was drawn.

The patients involved were drawn from a punch-card indexing system, and their subsequent history was extracted from case notes. A fuller description of method and procedure is

---

[1] On the other hand the immigration rate is also high (at about the same level as outward movement), so that the need for services in relation to the number of patients referred would probably be as great as in other areas where there was less migration. However, this would not be shown in the present study, in which mentally handicapped patients moving into Middlesex who have already been referred to another Local Authority are excluded.

given in Appendix 4, with a table showing the actual and the weighted number of subjects in the study.

FACTORS INFLUENCING REFERRAL RATES OVER THE PERIOD CONSIDERED

Before proceeding with a discussion of the numbers and rates of referrals of subnormal patients in Middlesex over the time period studied, it might be useful to consider what factors are likely to influence changes in referral rates in general. Referral rates may be influenced by any or all of the following factors: (1) the incidence of mental handicap; (2) the expectation of life of the mentally handicapped; (3) the system of referral; (4) the definition of a case.

(1) *Incidence*

There is no firm information on the incidence of mental handicap or on the way in which it may be changing, but suggestions can be made about the way in which different influences might be expected to act. Some examples are given below:

(a) *Severe mental handicap or low-grade defect.* (i) improved standards of living may reduce the rate of teratogenisis due to maternal malnutrition, both because fewer women will suffer from obstetrical abnormalities resulting from a poor diet in children and because fewer pregnant women will experience malnutrition (discussed as a cause by Crome, 1966);

(ii) improved ante-natal services and obstetrical procedures should reduce the incidence of certain malformations and birth-injury (Pasamanick and Lilienfeld, 1955);

(iii) the use of antibiotics and immunization should decrease the occurrence of abnormalities arising from common childhood illnesses such as measles;

(iv) on the other hand, not all conditions associated with mental handicap are related to poor social conditions and inadequate medical care (e.g. metabolic disorders and mongolism), and in these cases improved ante-natal and obstetrical services may increase the likelihood of malformed children being born alive. The example of certain neural tube defects is given in (2) below.

(b) *High-grade defect.* A certain proportion of high-grade defectives can be shown to suffer from organic pathology (Malamud, N., 1964). In the Local Health Authority series described here 20 per cent of feeble-minded and normal patients referred in 1959 and 1963 showed evidence of cerebral pathology (see pp 133–4). The incidence of these conditions will be influenced by the factors described above. It is likely, however, that in the majority of high-grade patients the I.Q. is depressed at least in part because they have experienced an unfavourable social and cultural environment. This view is supported by the disproportionate number of high-grade referrals who come from the lowest social classes and the poorest homes, and by the fact that improvement in I.Q. scores following special training in adolescence is correlated with poor socio-cultural conditions in the home. It would be expected on this evidence that as social conditions improve the incidence of high-grade defect would decline.

(2) *The expectation of life*
The increased use of antibiotics and the introduction of new surgical techniques are known to have prolonged the life-span of patients suffering from specific forms of mental handicap, for example mongols (Carter, C. O., 1958), and those with meningo-myeloceles (Mawdsley, *et al.*, 1967). Some of these patients formerly died before the age at which they would have been referred as handicapped, and their increased survival rates would have tended to increase referral rates. A possible paradigm of the conflicting ways in which different factors operate to influence administrative incidence is provided by figures of the incidence of spina bifida aperta and encephalocele in Birmingham (Leck, 1966). The incidence of the malformations shows some tendency to decline between 1950 and 1965 although subject to fluctuation. But over the same period still-births as a percentage of affected births fell from 24·4 to 20·5 and the percentage surviving for more than one year rose from 16·3 to 38·5. The majority of survivors will not be mentally handicapped (Mawdsley, *et al.*, op. cit), but the referral rate for mental handicap from this cause seems likely to increase.

(3) *The system of referral*

Improvements in the provision of care are likely to increase the number of cases referred. Thus the setting up of special care units for young children will make it worth while to refer a child of pre-school age as mentally handicapped, whereas before the existence of this facility there was little inducement to do so until the child reached school age. Young children are often known to the Health Department as mentally handicapped before they are formally notified, and in these cases it would be the responsibility of the clinic doctor or local medical officer to decide whether or not there was any purpose to be served by classifying the child as mentally handicapped at an early age. The pattern of his decision would affect rates of referral in the youngest age groups. Similarly the improvement in the services for adult patients which has occurred since the mid-1950s, in particular the increased number of places available in adult training-centres, may have encouraged parents or doctors to refer adult patients who as children were cared for privately. In addition, before 1959, referrals commonly involved formal legal ascertainment, and this possibly deterred a minority of families from bringing their relatives to the notice of the Local Health Authority. Since the 1959 Act, families may be more willing to refer their relatives than formerly.

(4) *The Definition of a case*

These are changes which may be closely allied to changes in the referral system. At one extreme a very inadequate system of referral might fail to cover people who by any criteria would be considered to be suffering from mental handicap. At the other, a very good system might cover most such people but explicitly exclude, for example, young children who also suffered from physical handicaps who were intentionally left to the care of another department.

There are many reasons, therefore, why rates of referral must be regarded as a poor guide to the incidence or prevalence of mental handicap. However, if one is interested, as we are here, in the changing demand for different kinds of services, changes in referral rates are of the utmost importance, regardless of whether a change in the true incidence of the condition has been demonstrated.

Age, grade and sex
Table 6.1 shows referrals for each year according to age and grade. Numbers of referrals rose by over 25 per cent between 1949 and the later years, although the population of Middlesex declined between the 1951 and 1961 censuses.

This increase occurred for all grades, except the very lowest, but it is particularly marked among the high-grade and normal referrals. After the 1959 Act, referral of high-grade patients to the Local Health Authority, when these patients left E.S.N. school was no longer statutory, as had previously been the case. In Middlesex, however, it was decided to refer all E.S.N. school-leavers, regardless of I.Q., to the Local Health Authority at 16 automatically, rather than select merely those thought to require further supervision. It was hoped in this way to keep a check on all these children for the first few years after they left school, in case they were in need of services. In consequence, in the later cohorts, there was a substantial increase in the number of high-grade and of normal referrals at the age of 16 years.

If the higher grades are omitted, however, there is only a small difference in the numbers referred, between the cohort years. In 1949 there was a higher number of patients whose grade could not be determined, because of insufficient information, than in the later cohort years, and in particular there were sixteen patients aged under 5 years of uncertain grade. It seems reasonable to assume that most of these were in fact severely mentally handicapped, since high-grade referrals in this age group are rare. In this case any difference over the increased tendency, in the later years, for lower-grade patients becomes almost negligible.

The only notable differences for the lower-grade patients over the time period studied are the slight increase in referrals of adult medium-grade patients, and the fact that there is an increased tendency, in the later years, for lower-grade children to be referred under the age of 5 years. The former probably reflects the longer life-expectancy of medium-grade patients, and the latter the improved techniques over the years for identifying mental handicap amongst young children.

In all three cohorts there were rather more males than

TABLE 6.1

AGE AND GRADE OF COHORTS OF REFERRALS TO MIDDLESEX COUNTY

Age groups	0–5	6–10	11–15	16	17–20	21–25	26–35	35+	Total	Per cent
1949										
Low-grade	10	12	2	0	0	0	0	0	24	9
Medium-grade	30	44	12	2	4	0	4	0	96	34
Low/medium-grade	14	0	0	0	0	0	0	0	14	5
High-grade	8	16	12	16	48	4	4	4	112	40
Normal	0	0	0	4	4	0	0	0	8	3
Grade not known	16	2	4	0	4	0	0	0	26	9
TOTAL	78	74	30	22	60	4	8	4	280	100·0
Per cent	28	26	11	8	21	1	3	1	100·0	100·0
1959										
Low-grade	14	0	0	0	0	0	0	0	34	4
Medium-grade	42	46	20	18	4	0	0	8	138	38
Low/medium-grade	2	0	0	0	0	0	0	0	2	—
High-grade	12	20	12	48	52	12	4	12	172	48
Normal	0	0	0	24	8	0	0	0	32	9
Grade not known	0	0	0	0	0	0	0	0	0	0
TOTAL	70	66	32	90	64	12	4	20	358	100·0
Per cent	19	18	9	25	18	3	1	5	100·0	100·0
1963										
Low-grade	18	2	0	0	0	0	0	0	20	6
Medium-grade	64	32	12	2	4	0	4	4	122	34
Low/medium-grade	10	2	2	0	0	0	0	4	18	5
High-grade	10	10	4	78	32	8	0	8	150	42
Normal	2	0	0	14	12	0	0	8	36	10
Grade not known	2	0	0	2	0	0	0	4	8	2
TOTAL	106	46	18	96	48	8	4	28	354	100·0
Per cent	30	13	5	27	13	2	1	8	100·0	100·0

females, as one would expect, but 1959 was peculiar in having a very high proportion of males (1949, 55 per cent; 1959, 63·1 per cent; 1963, 54 per cent).

Rates of Referral

More significant than changes in the *number* of referrals are any changes which appear in the referral *rate*, that is the number of mentally handicapped referred in relation to the size of the parent population, which is the population at risk. Overall, the referral rate increased over the period studied from 1·23 per 10,000 of the population at risk in 1949, to 1·6 per 10,000 in 1959 and 1·54 in 1963 (Table 6.2).

Rates for all age groups increased except for those patients aged between 6 and 15 years. Over the age of 25 years the number of referrals drops sharply as would be expected, but the rate of referral for this age group increased substantially in the later cohorts.

It should be borne in mind that the age-specific referral rates we quote are only approximate. The census years for which the age structure of the Middlesex population is known are two years removed from the period during which patients were referred. In that interval there may have been sufficient change in the population numbers in each age group to nullify some of the smaller changes in rates, but it seems unlikely that differences of more than 1·0 per ten thousand, or the direction of change, would be misleading. More important perhaps is the fact that the numbers in specific age and grade groups are small and therefore unreliable. These considerations limit the value of quoting age-specific rates by grade, and we do so primarily because they may be useful if other studies confirm the trends.

From a consideration of the numbers and rates of referrals, therefore, there is no reason to predict a decline in the demand for hospital care over the period studied; rather the reverse. There were no fewer low-grade children in the later years; there were slightly more adult low-grade patients and considerably more adult high-grade patients.

Referral rates for high-grade patients

The rate of referral for high-grade children (under the age of 15) remained approximately the same during the period

TABLE 6.2

PRIMARY REFERRAL RATES PER 10,000 POPULATION, BY COHORT

Age	Middlesex population 1951	1949 Mentally handicapped referred	Rate	Middlesex population 1961	1959 Mentally handicapped referred	Rate	1963 Mentally handicapped referred	Rate
0–5	175,088	78	4·45	151,210	70	4·62	106	7·01
6–10	157,451	74	4·70	131,934	66	5·00	46	3·48
11–15	137,576	30	2·18	161,960	32	1·97	18	1·11
16–25	273,488	86	3·14	303,314	166	5·47	152	5·01
26–35	328,013	8		284,413	4		4	
36–45	391,069	0		303,345	4		20	
46–55	340,840	0	0·08	357,654	12	0·19	0	0·26
56–65	237,345	4		285,091	4		8	
65+	228,445	0		255,622	0		0	
TOTAL	2,269,315	280	1·23	2,234,543	358	1·60	354	1·54

studied. However, the referral rate for those aged 16 years and over was much higher in the later cohort years, and it is this increase which is mainly responsible for the overall increased rate of referral. This seems largely to be due to the policy already noted of the routine referral of E.S.N. school-leavers. In 1949 rates of referral for high-grade patients, between 17 and 20 years, were higher than for those aged 16, which perhaps indicates less efficient detection of the potential problem group among these subjects in 1949, with referral occurring later when a crisis arose. On the other hand it is probable that many of the E.S.N. school-leavers in the later cohorts subsequently proved not to need services. Over the age of 25 years, about one-third of referrals were high-grade, and these also tended to increase in the later cohorts (see Table 6.3).

Referral rates for low-grade patients
There was a slight overall increase in the referral rate for severely mentally handicapped patients, but of a rather low order. This was partly due to a small but probably important increase in the rate of referral for adult medium-grade patients, possibly a result of improved life-expectancy for these patients. In the case of children the picture is not so clear, because of the number of patients in 1949 whose grade is uncertain, but it appears that there is a slight increase in the rate of referral of low- and medium-grade children, even if it is assumed that all of the 1949 'grade not known' children under 10 years are severely mentally handicapped (see Table 6.3).

Since it is known that the expectation of life of mongols has increased following the introduction of antibiotics (Carter, 1958), it seemed possible that the increase in the rate of referral of low-grade children was entirely due to this factor. Certainly the rate of referral for mongol patients did increase over the period studied (see Table 6.4), but there remained a slight, but very reduced, rise for even non-mongol patients between 1949 and 1963.

A further point to notice is that the rate of referral for the mentally handicapped under 5 years, primarily of low and medium grade, was much higher in 1963 (see Table 6.2), although the referral rate for severely mentally handicapped

E

TABLE 6.3

SUMMARY TABLE OF NUMBERS AND RATES OF REFERRAL

Approx I.Q	0–15 years	Rates per 10,000	16+ years	Rates per 10,000	Total	%	Rates per 10,000	25+ years	Rates per 10,000
1949 <50	124	2·63 (3·02)*	10	·06	134	(47·9)	·59 (·62)	4	·03
>50	36	·76	74	·53	110	(42·9)	·48	8	·06
Not known	22	—	4	—	26	(9·2)	—	—	—
TOTAL	182	3·87	88	·61	270	(100·0)	1·23	—	—
1959 <50	124	2·78	30	·19	154	(43·0)	·68	8	·06
>50	40	·98	160	1·04	204	(57·0)	·91	16	·13
Not known	0	—	0	—	0		—	—	—
TOTAL	164	3·69	190	1·23	358	(100·0)	1·60	—	—
1963 <50	142	3·19 (3·23)	18	·11	160	(45·7)	·71 (·72)	12	·09
>50	26	·58	160	1·04	186	(52·1)	·83	16	·13
Not known	2	—	6	—	8	(2·2)	—	—	—
TOTAL	170	3·73	184	1·19	354	(100·0)	1·59	—	—

* Figures in brackets in column 2 give rates per 10,000 assuming that all the 'grade not known' admissions under the age of 10 years have an I.Q. under 50.

TABLE 6.4

REFERRAL RATES FOR SEVERELY MENTALLY HANDICAPPED PATIENTS,
MONGOLS AND NON-MONGOLS SEPARATELY

	1949		1959		1965	
	Number	*Rate per* 10,000	*Number*	*Rate per* 10,000	*Number*	*Rate per* 10,000
<10 years	128*	3·84	104	3·67	130	4·58
Mongols	36	1·08	52	1·83	38	1·34
Non-mongols	92	2·76	52	1·83	92	3·24
<15 years	142*	3·02	124	2·78	142	3·19
Mongols	38	0·80	58	1·30	40	·90
Non-mongols	104	2·22	66	1·48	104	

* The 1949 figures assume that the eighteen 'grade not known'
patients under the age of 10 years are all severely subnormal.

patients under 15 years increased only slightly (see Table 6.3).
This suggests that the system for identifying severe mental
handicap had improved, so that by 1963 many more of these
cases came to light in the pre-school period than in 1949. The
slightly increased rate of referral for low-grade children, therefore, is probably due more to improved and earlier detection
of cases in the later years than to any increase in the incidence
or prevalence of mental handicap.

Source of referrals
This information was fairly complete for all three cohorts, the
majority of referrals being made under Section 3 or Section 5
of the Education Act. Section 3 of the Education Act refers
to children found unable to cope within the normal school
system (usually they are from E.S.N. schools) who, therefore,
were transferred to Local Health Authority training-centres
to complete their education. The proportion referred in this
way declined over the period studied, and again this indicates
better detection of cases within the pre-school period. Section 5
of the Act covers referrals made at 16 as children leave E.S.N.
schools. These increased between 1949 and 1963, as we have
already described (see Table 6.5).

Diagnosis
Between about one-fifth and one-quarter of the referrals for
each year were given a definite diagnosis. In each cohort most

TABLE 6.5

SOURCE OF REFERRAL FOR MIDDLESEX PATIENTS

	1949		1959		1963	
	N	%	N	%	N	%
Hospital	50	(17·9)	34	(19·5)	64	(18·1)
Education Sect. 3	90	(32·1)	90	(25·3)	54	(15·2)
Education Sect. 5	48	(17·0)	122	(42·7)	110	(31·1)
Police	12	—	8	—	4	—
Other	62	(22·1)	94	(16·3)	112	(31·6)
Not known	18	—	10	—	10	—
Total	280	(100·0)	358	(100·0)	354	(100·0)

of these patients were mongols. Using other information on the case-notes which was of possible aetiological significance as well as the actual diagnosis, it was possible to assign a larger number of patients to the positive diagnostic categories devised by Heber (1961). This reveals an upward trend in the conditions attributed to the effects of infection, intoxication or injury (from 6 to 18 per cent). This is probably due to improved record-taking and the greater availability of information from paediatric and general hospitals for the later years, and parallels the reduction in the number of 'not knowns' from 47 to 32 per cent. In all three years most of the patients classified in these terms were under 15 years of age on referral, and most of those were less than 5 years old.

OTHER CHARACTERISTICS OF THE COHORTS

Ideally it would be useful to make comparisons between cohorts for characteristics such as sensory and motor handicap, epilepsy, brain damage or emotional disorders, since changes in the percentage of patients with these problems might affect demand for residential services. However the data available on the 1949 cohort was often very poor, and for most characteristics recorded there was insufficient information to classify between 20 per cent and 30 per cent of cases. This invalidates comparison, and the most that can be said is that there is no evidence that rates for physical or emotional handicaps were higher in 1949 than in the later cohorts.

Dependency

Patients were first rated on a scale of independence. The points on the scale were 'completely dependent', 'partly dependent' and 'independent'.[2]

In 1959 and 1963 between one-fifth and one-quarter of referrals were completely or almost completely helpless. At least 70 per cent in both cohorts were either wholly or almost wholly independent. If the 'unknowns' in 1949 were distributed equally throughout the scale, there would be a similar proportion of helpless and independent patients at that time also (see Table 6.6).

TABLE 6.6

PERCENTAGE OF INDEPENDENT AND DEPENDENT PATIENTS IN EACH COHORT

	1949	1959	1963
Completely dependent	17	21	23
Partly dependent	6	8	7
Independent	50	63	59
Not known	27	8	11
TOTAL	100	100	100

Physical handicap

Between 40 and 45 per cent of all patients in the two cohorts had some physical handicap which would be considered a problem even in a person of normal intelligence, and so constitutes a significant handicap over and above poor intellectual ability (see Table 6.7). This is usually a motor or sensory handicap or epilepsy, but the category also includes a few cases with problems such as hydrocephaly or syndactyly.

In the later cohorts between 12 and 17 per cent of patients had a sensory handicap, blindness being noted more frequently than deafness (see Table 6.7). Between 16 per cent and 21 per cent of referrals showed a motor dysfunction, the majority of these being attributed to cerebral palsy. About 20 per cent were or had been epileptic at some point in their lives.

Brain damage

Taking together all gross physical signs and conditions which indicate the likelihood of damage to brain tissue, about a third

[2] The method of rating this and other attributes is described in Appendix 4.

TABLE 6.7

PHYSICAL HANDICAP AMONG COHORTS OF REFERRALS

	1949 %	1959 %	1963 %
Some handicap	34	39	45
Any motor handicap	11	16	21
(Cerebral palsy)	(7)	(15)	(17)
Epilepsy	15	23	20
Sensory handicap	5	12	17
Blind	4	6	10
Deaf	1	4	5
Both	0	2	2

of each of the later cohorts showed some signs of brain damage (between 80 per cent and 100 per cent of low-grade patients and between 36 and 46 per cent of medium-grade patients). This is to be expected since it is known that most idiots and many imbeciles show evidence of brain abnormalities on autopsy (Crome, 1966, Malamud, 1966). However, in the later cohorts where reporting was fairly good, 20 per cent of even the high-grade and normal patients appeared to be brain-damaged.

Intelligence

Again, reporting is much more complete in the later cohorts. Less than 35 per cent in the two later cohorts had no I.Q. recorded, compared with nearly 60 per cent in 1949. Very few in any cohort who were not tested soon after referral (within two years) were tested subsequently. Although it is possible that assessments were made at the training-centres which were never recorded in the case-notes.

It is of interest that in 1959 and 1963 about 40 per cent of reported cases had I.Q.s over 50 and that 10 per cent had I.Q.s within the normal range, i.e. over 70. This is primarily due to the large number of E.S.N. school-leavers referred under Section 57/5 of the Education Act. As might be expected, the I.Q. of those referred in the younger age group is lower than for those referred later, but there are substantial numbers with I.Q.s over 50 reported before the age of 16 (N = 40 in 1959; N = 26 in 1963).

Speech

It was not possible to assess degree of speech from the information in the case-notes, but use of speech was usually noted, so in this study 'speaking' merely means the ability to use at least single words. A rather smaller number of patients would have useful speech (i.e. ability to make their common needs known or use sentences).

Between a half and two-thirds of each cohort was able to uses some speech, and virtually everyone over the age of 16 could speak in all three cohorts. In 1959 and 1963, where information was very complete, about 90 per cent of those over the age of 10 could speak.

Behaviour disturbances

In each cohort about the same proportion, between 30 and 40 per cent, were recorded as having some behaviour disturbance. About a quarter of these showed a neurotic or psychotic disturbance, and the rest were primarily conduct disorders. Thirty-seven per cent of those patients who were low-grade and 40 per cent of the high-grade patients had some behaviour disorder; the highest percentage being in the 'normal' group and the next highest in the 'imbecile' group. Some disorders were more characteristic of the the low-grade patients, namely screaming, self-injury, hyperactivity or restlessness. Other disorders, such as psychosis, neurosis, delinquency and psychopathy were more common among high-grade patients. Aggression, destructiveness, and minor conduct disorders were found in all grades, although the kind of behaviour involved was probably very different.

For all grades and all cohorts, more young patients were reported to have a behaviour disorder, even allowing for the fact that more of the referrals are in the younger age group (34 per cent of those under 16 were reported as having a behaviour disorder, but only 29 per cent of those aged 16 years or more). Disorders in the younger age groups were mainly of the kind characteristic of 'low-grade' patients.

There were no marked differences between cohorts, except that rather more neurotic and minor conduct disorders were noted in the later years, which may well be due simply to better reporting. There was also an increase in the number with autistic or schizophrenic behaviour reported, which may indicate a greater willingness to recognize the possibility of these conditions among mentally handicapped patients.

SUMMARY

In general therefore the major differences found between cohorts can be summarized as follows :

(a) There was an increase in the number of high-grade patients referred over the age of 16 years.

(b) There was a small increase in the number of adult medium-grade patients referred.

(c) There was a very slight, possibly negligible, increase in the number of low-grade children referred.

(d) It was not possible to make valid comparison between 1949 and the later cohorts with regard to handicap, but there was no evidence for any increase in the amount of handicap between the years studied, quite similar proportions being dependent, physically handicapped or emotionally disturbed.

Accordingly it seems unlikely that any differences in the services Middlesex patients experienced could be attributed to any great extent to changes in the characteristics of the patients, perhaps with the exception of the need to cater for more high-grade patients. Certainly one would not expect from the data discussed above that the demand for hospital care would have declined over the period studied; and, if anything, from this evidence alone it might have been expected to have increased.

PATIENTS' EXPERIENCE OF CARE AFTER REFERRAL

In Chapter 5 we showed how, although the numbers of patients first admitted to hospital had greatly increased since 1949, the number of long-term admissions had dropped and the proportions remaining in hospital at successive intervals after admission had decreased. Similarly, the proportions of the Middlesex patients who were in long-term hospital care at any period following referral in 1959 and 1963 were much lower

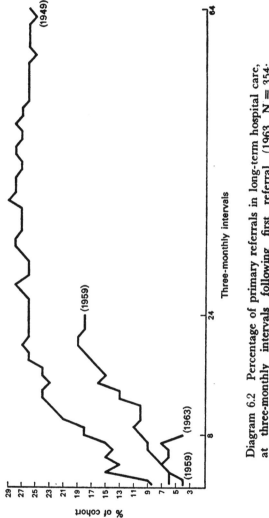

Diagram 6.2 Percentage of primary referrals in long-term hospital care, at three-monthly intervals following first referral (1963 N = 354; 1959 N = 358; 1949 N = 280)

than the percentage of patients in hospital at corresponding intervals after referral in 1949 (Diagram 6.2).[3]

The decline in the proportion of successive cohorts in hospital occurred in each grade but was least marked for low-grade patients. It affected every age group (see diagram), but we shall concentrate on those who were less than 5 years old at referral, and those aged from 15 up to 20 years. These groups contained the greatest numbers of patients, but they differed widely in many characteristics besides age. Those under 5 years contained a higher proportion of low-grade patients than any other age group, particularly in the later years when virtually all the low-grade were referred before the age of 5. By contrast, the majority of referrals in the 15- to 20-year group had an I.Q. of over 50, and none was low-grade. The younger group also contained many more patients with physical handicaps of all kinds than did those referred between 15 and 20 years. In the hospital cohort study described in Chapter 5, admissions in these age groups were more frequent than in any other five-year group, and so both groups are likely to be highly at risk for hospital admission, though for very different reasons.

For children referred under the age of 5 there were successive declines in the proportions of each cohort to be found in hospital at each three-monthly interval following referral (see Diagram 6.3a). For those referred between 15 and 20 years there was a considerable fall between 1949 and 1959, but a small and not compensatory increase for patients referred in 1963 (Diagram 6.3b). There are two possible explanations for this decline: either the demand for hospital care fell during the period, or a greater proportion of demand remained unsatisfied in the later cohorts. If demand fell this could have been due to a higher rate of depletion in the later cohorts (by death, discharge or emigration) rather than to any increase in the provision of other forms of residential care, or to an increase in non-residential community care. We shall consider each of these possibilities in turn.

[3] In this section we are considering long-term care when discussing hospital admissions. This is because we are no longer primarily considering the burden on the hospitals, but rather the patterns of community services which parallel changes in the demand for hospital care. From this point of view short-term care can be considered as part of the community services.

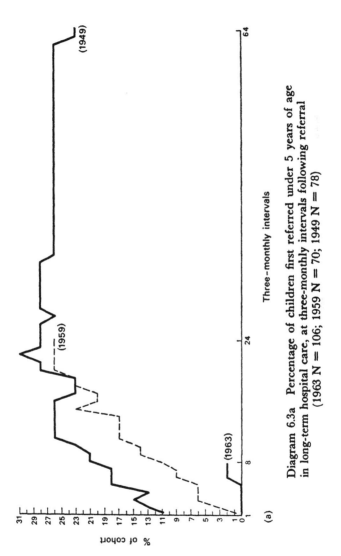

Diagram 6.3a Percentage of children first referred under 5 years of age in long-term hospital care, at three-monthly intervals following referral (1963 N = 106; 1959 N = 70; 1949 N = 78)

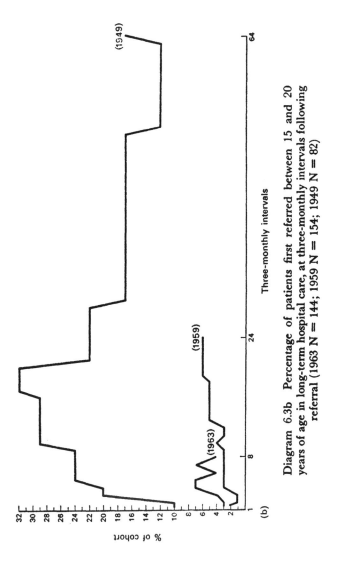

Diagram 6.3b   Percentage of patients first referred between 15 and 20 years of age in long-term hospital care, at three-monthly intervals following referral (1963 N = 144; 1959 N = 154; 1949 N = 82)

The demand for hospital care

Demand for residential care is defined here as the sum of patients in long-term hospital care together with those on the waiting-list. The Middlesex Health Authority kept a waiting-list of patients in need of hospital care, which appeared to be comprehensive and to include all those patients whose relatives expressed a wish for them to be in hospital. Of course it is impossible to determine from case records whether any relatives were discouraged from asking for hospital admission, or whether any such requests were unrecorded, but in all cases where the wish *was* recorded the patient was placed on the waiting-list, and remained there until he or she entered hospital or died, or the relatives decided to keep him at home.

Diagram 6.4 shows the proportion of each original cohort demanding hospital care at three-monthly intervals following referral. The decline in demand for hospital care was even more marked between the three cohorts than the fall in the proportion in hospital. For very young children (under 5 years) there was no decline in demand between 1949 and 1959 until more than two years after referral, but a dramatic fall between the latter year and 1963 (see Diagram 6.5a). The pattern for young adults (15–20 years) was almost identical with their experience of hospital care (i.e. a drop between 1949 and 1959 and little change thereafter) and this was because very few of these patients were on a waiting-list – the waiting-lists for all three cohorts being almost exclusively composed of children referred before the age of 10 (Diagram 6.5b).[4]

Death, discharge and emigration

The later cohorts show a small increase in depletion rates compared with those referred in 1949 (Diagram 6.6) and this could account for some of the decline in demand. However, considering first the young children, *smaller* proportions of the later cohort were lost through death, discharge and emigration from the area, and therefore the *potential* demand for hospital care amongst these patients was actually greater in 1959 and 1963 than in 1949 (Diagram 6.7a). The lower depletion rate in the later years for the under-fives was due to

---

[4] This result ties in with Leeson's finding that few high-grade adolescents were admitted from a waiting-list, most being 'crisis' admissions following some social breakdown in the patient or his family (Leeson, 1963).

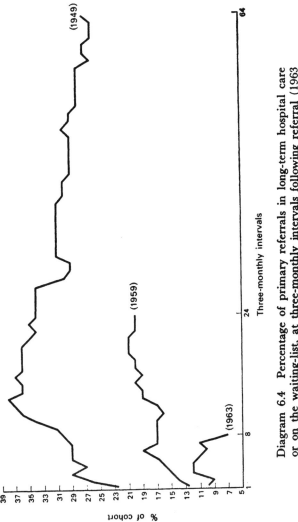

Diagram 6.4   Percentage of primary referrals in long-term hospital care or on the waiting-list, at three-monthly intervals following referral (1963 N = 354; 1959 N = 358; 1959 N = 280)

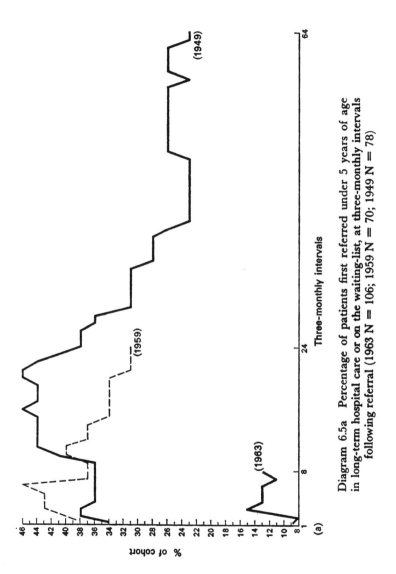

Diagram 6.5a Percentage of patients first referred under 5 years of age in long-term hospital care or on the waiting-list, at three-monthly intervals following referral (1963 N = 106; 1959 N = 70; 1949 N = 78)

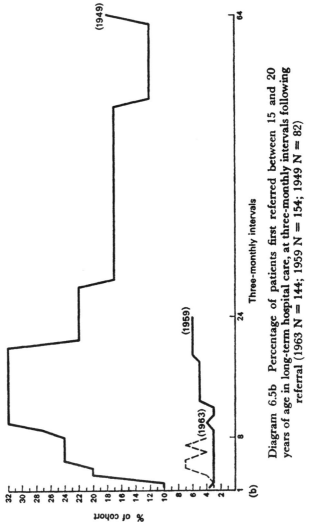

Diagram 6.5b   Percentage of patients first referred between 15 and 20 years of age in long-term hospital care, at three-monthly intervals following referral (1963 N = 144; 1959 N = 154; 1949 N = 82)

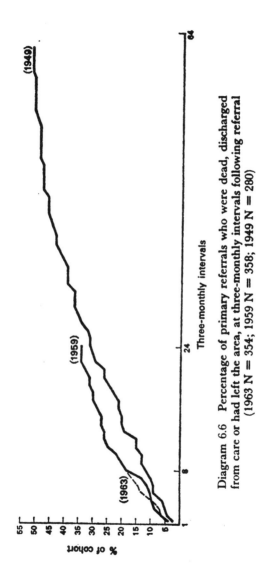

Diagram 6.6   Percentage of primary referrals who were dead, discharged from care or had left the area, at three-monthly intervals following referral (1963 N = 354; 1959 N = 358; 1949 N = 280)

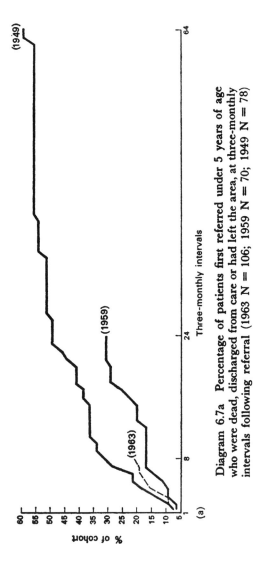

Diagram 6.7a Percentage of patients first referred under 5 years of age who were dead, discharged from care or had left the area, at three-monthly intervals following referral (1963 N = 106; 1959 N = 70; 1949 N = 78)

small decreases in the death and emigration rates although, as was to be expected, the death rate for these patients was higher than for any other age group in all three cohorts.

By contrast the increased depletion rates for the 15 to 20-year-olds was mainly the result of increased emigration from the area during the first two years following referral, and thereafter to an increased rate of discharge (see Diagram 6.7b). Nearly all discharges recorded occurred among patients of this age group, being mainly high-grade patients who were referred after leaving E.S.N. schools but showed after a short period of surveillance that they were able to cope without supervision. Proof of this consisted of holding down a job or getting married.

There was little evidence that children referred early (before 15 years) were later able to be discharged or to live independently. Only one child referred between 10 and 15 years in 1949, and one of those referred under 15 years in 1959 or 1963, was discharged as an adolescent or adult. However in the later cohorts only those aged between 10 and 15 could have reached the age of employment or marriage at follow-up, and it is too early to say whether or not the early training received by the 1959 and 1963 patients has increased the proportion of subnormals who can later live as independent adults.

The demand for all residential care
Since the rise in depletion rates alone could not account for the declining demand for hospital care, it seemed probable that the provision of alternative forms of care did so. The first possibility here was that alternative forms of residential care had been provided. Local authorities have been encouraged in the last decade to provide accommodation for patients other than full hospital care. In Middlesex this included foster care and guardianship, hostel residence and short-term hospital care.

Foster care consisted either of care similar to that provided for normal children, where the child is placed with a private family, or placement in a small private residential home which took a number of similar young people. Hostel care was used for high- and medium-grade patients who were capable at least of working. Short-term care has already been described in the previous chapter. In Middlesex it was used greatly for patients already on the waiting-list (in 1959 and 1963 nearly 50 per cent of short-term admissions were for patients already

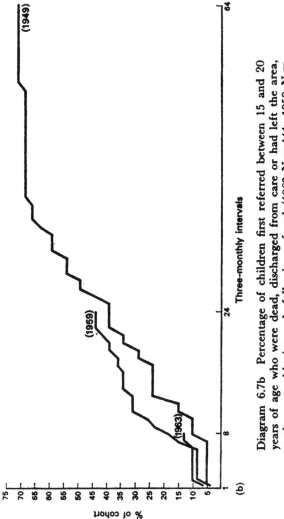

Diagram 6.7b Percentage of children first referred between 15 and 20 years of age who were dead, discharged from care or had left the area, at three-monthly intervals following referral (1963 N = 144; 1959 N = 154; 1949 N = 82)

on the waiting-list) but could also be provided to enable families, willing to keep the patient at home, to take a holiday or a rest.

The demand for residential care, therefore, is here defined as all patients in hospital, for short- or long-term care, or resident in hostels or foster homes, together with those on the waiting-list for any form of residential care. Diagram 6.8 shows that demand for residential care declined between 1949 and 1959, but that there was very little difference between 1959 and 1963. The patterns both for children referred before the age of 5 years and for the 15 to 20-year group were similar to the patterns already described for hospital demand, although the difference between the early and later cohorts was rather less (Diagrams 6.9a and b). This was because of a small rise in the provision of extra-hospital residential care which was particularly marked for these age groups.

Training
If the increased accommodation in the community played some part in reducing the demand for hospital care, it was a small one, and it would appear therefore that the overall demand for residential care did indeed decline over the period studied. The most obvious change accompanying the declining demand was an increase in the proportions of the successive cohorts receiving training in the community.

In Middlesex, as in most areas, training-centres were provided both for children under 16 who received social training and education, and for older patients who were engaged in industrial contract work or were working under special supervision in factories. In addition, from 1957 special care units were provided for the very young or very handicapped who could not be contained within junior training centres.

Diagram 6.10 shows the percentage of patients referred in each year who were in training-centres or special care units at the end of threemonthly intervals following referral. The percentage receiving training shows a progressive increase between the three cohorts, and this increase was most clearly marked for those aged under 5 years and those aged between 15 and 20 years, at the time of referral. In fact in 1949 there was no provision at all for young adults until more than five years after referral, whereas of the 1963 cohort 25 per cent were

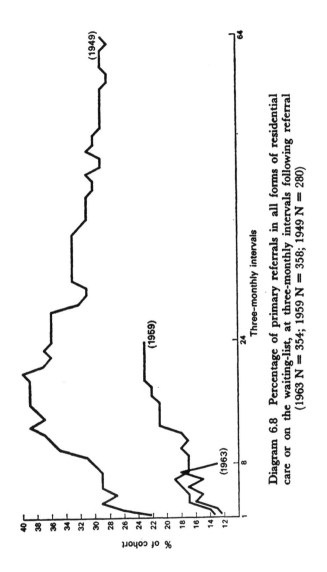

Diagram 6.8 Percentage of primary referrals in all forms of residential care or on the waiting-list, at three-monthly intervals following referral (1963 N = 354; 1959 N = 358; 1949 N = 280)

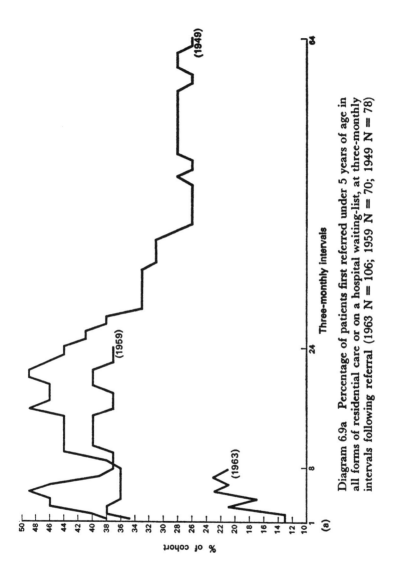

Diagram 6.9a Percentage of patients first referred under 5 years of age in all forms of residential care or on a hospital waiting-list, at three-monthly intervals following referral (1963 N = 106; 1959 N = 70; 1949 N = 78)

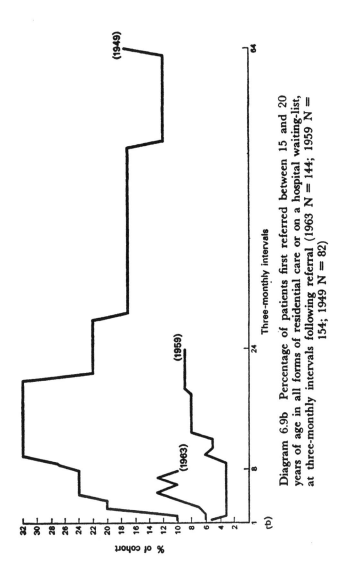

Diagram 6.9b Percentage of patients first referred between 15 and 20 years of age in all forms of residential care or on a hospital waiting-list, at three-monthly intervals following referral (1963 N = 144; 1959 N = 154; 1949 N = 82)

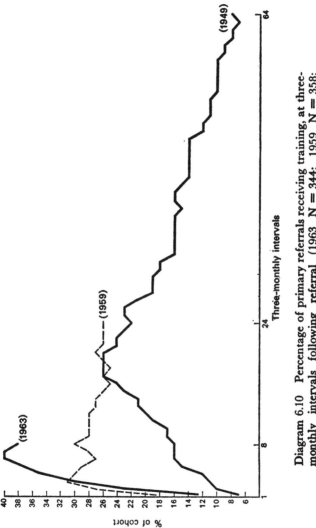

Diagram 6.10 Percentage of primary referrals receiving training, at three-monthly intervals following referral (1963 N = 344; 1959 N = 358; 1949 N = 280)

receiving training within two years of referral. On the other hand there was little difference between 1959 and 1963 in the percentage of this age group receiving training (Diagrams 6.11a and b). It will be remembered that, parallel to this, there was a drop in the demand for hospital care for this group between 1949 and 1959, at the same time as the increase in training occurred, but little alteration in the volume of demand between the two later cohorts. Considering the case of children, that is all patients referred under the age of 15, in 1949 only 28 per cent were receiving training, whereas by 1963 almost all who were available (i.e. alive and in Middlesex) were receiving training within two years of referral. Therefore, for this age group, also, the expansion of training-centre places paralleled the decline in demand for hospital care. In particular, with the development of special care units, the percentage of children under 5 years of age receiving training expanded enormously, so that while only 4 per cent of this age group were in training in 1949, 60 per cent of the 1963 cohort were receiving at least part-time training. It was for this group perhaps above all that training-centre provision appeared to effect a change in the demand for hospital care.[5]

The position of all patients referred in each of the three cohorts is summarized in Tables 6.8a b, c. There is good evidence here to support the proposition that an increase in the provision of training in the community results in a decline in the demand for hospital care. The clear implication is that any Local Health Authority able to support the high rate of community care which Middlesex latterly provided could expect to see a similar fall in the immediate demand for hospital care.

Some questions, however, remain unanswered. One is: why was there little difference between 1959 and 1963 in the pattern of care for young adults? Many people in these age groups were employed, particularly amongst those referred in later cohorts. It was shown earlier in this chapter that there was a considerable increase over the period studied in the numbers of patients of these ages referred on leaving E.S.N. schools, and we suggested that some of these were likely to need only

---

[5] Doubtless the provision of short-term hospital care for this age group also contributed to the change in demand for long-term care, and this will be discussed in the following section.

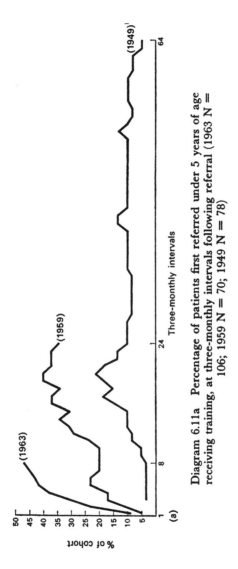

Diagram 6.11a Percentage of patients first referred under 5 years of age receiving training, at three-monthly intervals following referral (1963 N = 106; 1959 N = 70; 1949 N = 78)

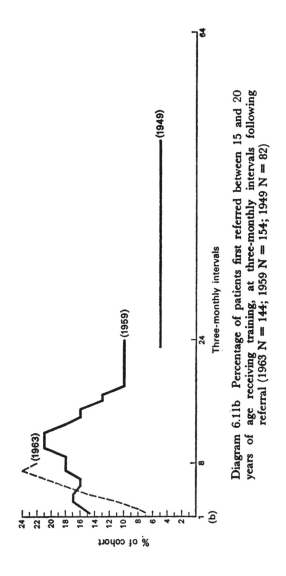

Diagram 6.11b Percentage of patients first referred between 15 and 20 years of age receiving training, at three-monthly intervals following referral (1963 N = 144; 1959 N = 154; 1949 N = 82)

TABLE 6.8a

PATIENTS' EXPERIENCE OF CARE 2 YEARS AFTER REFERRAL, BY AGE AND COHORT

Age groups	0–5		6–10		11–15		16–20		20+		Total	
	N	%	N	%	N	%	N	%	N	%	N	%
1949												
Initial cohort	78	100	74	100	30	100	82	100	16	100	280	100
Dead	10	13	—	—	2	7	—	—	—	—	34	12
Discharged	2	3	—	—	—	—	4	5	—	—	}	
Left area, etc.	12	15	—	—	—	—	4	5	—	—		
Total remaining	54	100	74	100	28	100	74	100	16	100	246	100
In L.T. hospital	16	30	6	8	4	14	20	27	4	25	50	20
In other res. care	—	—	—	—	—	—	—	—	—	—	—	—
Training-centres	2	4	30	41	12	43	—	—	—	—	44	18
Working	—	—	—	—	—	—	16	22	—	—	16	7
Total accounted for	18	33	36	49	16	57	36	49	4	25	110	45
(Waiting-list)	(12)	(22)	(18)	(24)	(—)	(—)	(—)	(—)	(4)	(25)	(34)	(14)
1959												
Initial cohort	70	100	66	100	32	100	154	100	36	100	358	100
Dead	8	11	—	—	—	—	—	—	—	—	64	18
Discharged	—	—	6	9	2	6	12	8	—	—	}	
Left area, etc.	4	6	8	12	—	—	16	10	8	22		
Total remaining	58	100	52	100	30	100	126	100	28	100	294	100
In L.T. hospital	8	14	2	4	6	20	4	3	16	57	36	12
In other res. care	6	10	—	—	—	—	—	—	—	—	6	2
Training-centres	14	24	36	69	20	67	28	22	8	28	106	36
Working	—	—	—	—	—	—	74	59	—	—	74	25
Total accounted for	28	48	38	73	26	87	106	84	24	86	222	76
(Waiting-list)	(18)	(31)	(6)	(12)	(—)	(—)	(—)	(—)	(—)	(—)	(24)	(8)

TABLE 6.8a—continued

Age groups	0–5 N	0–5 %	6–10 N	6–10 %	11–15 N	11–15 %	16–20 N	16–20 %	20+ N	20+ %	Total N	Total %
1963												
Initial cohort	106	100	46	100	18	100	144	100	40	100	354	100
Dead	8	8	2	4	—	—	4	3	4	10 }	64	18 }
Discharged	4	4	—	—	—	—	14	10	12	30		
Left area, etc.	10	9	4	9	2	11						
Total remaining	84	100	40	100	16	100	126	100	24	100	290	100
In L.T. hospital	2	2	2	5	—	—	6	5	4	17	14	5
In other res. care	10	12	—	—	—	—	8	6	4	17	22	8
Training-centres	50	60	38	95	12	75	32	25	4	17	136	47
Working	—	—	—	—	—	—	60	48	—	—	60	21
Total accounted for	62	74	40	100	12	75	106	84	12	50	232	80
(Waiting-list)	(12)	(14)	(—)	(—)	(—)	(—)	(—)	(—)	(—)	(—)	(12)	(4)

Note: On this and the following two tables 'other residential care' is added to the other items to give 'Total accounted for'. This is not strictly correct since a few patients in other residential care are also in training-centres or working.

TABLE 6.8(b)

PATIENTS' EXPERIENCE 6 YEARS AFTER REFERRAL

	0–5 N	0–5 %	6–10 N	6–10 %	11–15 N	11–15 %	16–20 N	16–20 %	20+ N	20+ %	Total N	Total %
1949												
Initial cohort	78	100	74	100	30	100	82	100	16	100	280	100
Dead	18	23	4	5	4	13	—	—	—	— }	86	31 }
Discharged	4	5	—	—	—	—	16	20	4	25		
Left area, etc.	16	21	4	5	—	—	16	20	12	25		
Total remaining	40	100	66	100	26	100	50	100	4	100	194	100
In L.T. hospital	22	55	22	33	8	31	18	36	4	33	74	38
In other res. care	2	5	4	6	2	8	—	—	—	—	8	4
Training-centres	8	20	38	58	12	46	12	24	—	—	62	32
Working	—	—	—	—	2	8	2	8	—	—	14	7
Total accounted for	32	80	64	97	24	92	34	68	4	33	158	81
(Waiting-list)	(8)	(20)	(12)	(18)	(2)	(8)	(—)	(—)	(—)	(—)	(22)	(11)

TABLE 6.8b—continued

Age groups

1959	0–5 N	0–5 %	6–10 N	6–10 %	11–15 N	11–15 %	16–20 N	16–20 %	20+ N	20+ %	Total N	Total %
Initial cohort	70	100	66	100	32	100	154	100	36	100	358	100
Dead	14	20	2	3	—	—	—	—	4	11	}	}
Discharged	2	3	6	9	—	—	40	26	—	—	122	34
Left area, etc.	6	9	8	12	4	12	28	18	8	22	}	}
Total remaining	48	100	50	100	28	100	86	100	24	100	236	100
In L.T. hospital	18	37	12	24	8	28	10	11	16	67	64	27
In other res. care	6	13	—	—	—	—	4	5	4	17	14	6
Training-centres	24	50	34	68	14	50	16	19	—	—	88	37
Working	—	—	—	—	—	—	50	58	4	17	54	23
Total accounted for	48	100	46	92	22	79	80	93	24	100	220	93
(Waiting-list)	(4)	(8)	(2)	(4)	(—)	(—)	(—)	(—)	(—)	(—)	(6)	(3)

TABLE 6.8(c)

PATIENTS' EXPERIENCE 16 YEARS AFTER REFERRAL

1949	0–5 N	0–5 %	6–10 N	6–10 %	11–15 N	11–15 %	16–20 N	16–20 %	20+ N	20+ %	Total N	Total %
Initial cohort	78	100	74	100	30	100	82	100	16	100	280	100
Dead	26	33	12	16	4	13	4	5	4	25	}	}
Discharged	4	5	—	—	2	7	28	34	—	—	150	54
Left Area, etc.	16	21	16	22	4	13	26	32	4	25	}	}
Total remaining	32	100	46	100	20	100	24	100	8	100	130	100
In L.T. hospital	18	56	28	61	10	50	14	58	4	50	74	57
In other res. care	2	6	2	4	2	10	—	—	—	—	6	5
Training-centres	4	12	12	26	6	30	—	—	—	—	22	17
Working	—	—	4	9	—	—	10	42	—	—	14	11
Total accounted for	24	75	46	100	18	90	24	100	4	50	116	89
(Waiting-list)	(—)	(—)	(2)	(4)	(—)	(—)	(—)	(—)	(—)	(—)	(2)	(2)

minimal supervision. The fact that so many of them were able to work (about half of the 1959 and 1963 referrals in this age group were in employment within two years of referral) is an indication of their social competence. However even in 1963 some 16 per cent were neither working nor receiving any form of care, and between 3 per cent and 5 per cent were in hospitals. The proportion in hospital changed very little between 1959 and 1963. The actual numbers in hospital, of course, were very small, but this is likely to be a reliable result, since the same pattern was evident in the hospital cohort study described in the previous chapter. The most likely explanation is that the optimum level of training of the kind then given had been provided for this group by 1959, and that thereafter the proportion entering hospital fluctuated with chance variations in the proportion who were handicapped by physical or behavioural abnormalities. If this is true, then a further reduction in hospital demand could perhaps be brought about, but only by the provision of modes of community care different from those at present available – for example, different kinds of training programmes or hostel placement. Intensive studies of these patients and their families are needed in order to throw light on this issue.

A second problem concerns the youngest patients. There was a clear and progressive reduction in the demand for residential care at the time when an increasing proportion were provided with training. But at the time of follow-up the oldest of the group referred in 1959 were less than 11 years old. What will happen when these patients reach adulthood? Most of the attention in recent years has been focused on provision for children, but if they cannot be retained in the community when they grow up it may be asked, among other things, whether their families should have been encouraged to accept for so long the sacrifices which caring for a severely handicapped child entails, even when adequate training is provided. The question has been well discussed by Fryers and Mountriey (1965). It may of course turn out that a high proportion of the surviving children are able to remain at home until their parents die or become too elderly to care for them, but as yet we do not know; this is a problem which requires an answer as early as possible. This is not only because of the moral questions which are involved, but also because the type of care and training which these children receive in the community should bear some relationship to their future prospects. Perhaps the development of community residential care on a weekly basis, which is envisaged as part of the Wessex experiment, might help both the child and his parents to accommodate to the immediate and long-term problems of care for severely mentally handicapped patients.

Short-term care

Only passing attention has been given to this facility in the present chapter so far. This is because the emphasis here has been on the variables responsible for the decline in long-term hospital care, and it is not possible by the method used to assess the effects of short-term care on the demand for long-term placement. This is because, after the first admission, short-term hospital care forms only a tiny proportion of total hospital care for each cohort of referrals.

However, as we showed in the previous chapter, the volume of short-term admissions increased enormously over the period studied, and this provision certainly must have had a greatly beneficial effect on the families involved. Half of the short-stay admissions from the Local Health Authority cohorts were drawn from patients already on the waiting-list for long-term admission, so that this service was used to a large extent to help families who had already decided that they could not cope with their mentally handicapped relatives at home. There is no way of assessing this point, but perhaps the knowledge that regular relief was available may have had the effect of lessening pressure from these families for immediate long-term hospital care. Even during the brief follow-up period available in this study, however, a number of patients admitted initially in 1959 and 1963 as short-stay cases were retained or re-admitted on a permanent basis, and at best this facility is likely to postpone rather than to stem demand in real cases of need. However, in combination with special care unit places for the under-fives, this service may have helped to reduce demand for young children at least while the child was still small enough to be handled easily at home.

CONCLUSIONS

Over the period studied referral rates increased for all types of patient but particularly for high-grade adolescents and

F

medium-grade adults. At the same time the number of admissions to hospital declined, and although this decline was accompanied by the development of community residential care, the number of residential places available outside the hospital service were very few and insufficient to make much impact on the numbers admitted to long-term residential care. Furthermore the percentage of patients on the waiting-list also declined, so that a genuine decline in the demand for long-term residential care seems to have occurred. The only changes in the pattern of community services of sufficient order to account for this are, in the first place, the increase in training facilities, and secondly, the development of a system of short-term care.

It is not possible by the cohort method to calculate the effect of the latter policy on demand for long-term residential care, but we suggest that it has played a part in reducing pressure on hospital beds, over the short run. However, the investigation of the relationship between the expansion of training for particular age groups and the changing pattern of demand for hospital care clearly indicates that there is a strong correlation between the two.

Since training facilities in Middlesex expanded at a faster rate than throughout the country generally, it may be assumed that the same pattern of change will occur in other areas as the level of community training increases. Although there was some indication from this study that community residential services affected hospital placement, even in Middlesex this service was in its infancy at the time of the follow-up. However, the evidence does suggest that hospital or other residential facilities within the community can reduce pressure on hospital beds, and perhaps for high-grade patients this is the only development which can substantially affect the demand for hospital care in an area where training facilities are adequate.

Considerations which cannot be fully registered in a purely statistical study are the real feelings and wishes of patients and their families with regard to services. A study which followed the 'natural history' of patient handicap and the problems encountered by their families would yield much useful information about the kind of provision which should be made in the future, and would provide a measure of 'consumer appreciation' which is unfortunately lacking when assessing the effects of most of the social services. Previous work in other areas (Tizard and Grad, 1961; Moncrieffe, 1966) does show that families on the whole wish to care themselves for their mentally handicapped members for as long as they can. But we must surely hesitate to encourage them to do so without ensuring that adequate support is available, and the same authors clearly showed how poor this is in many respects.

Finally, although we can see from this study that the need for hospital care can be reduced if community services are improved, there was still a waiting-list for hospital beds at the end of the follow-up, and some of the families involved were obliged to keep their mentally handicapped relatives at home long after the situation became really difficult for them. While some workers have suggested that a more active discharge policy coupled with a policy of opening more long-term residential hostels could reduce the number of patients in hospital (Leck, *et al.*, 1967), there is an obvious need for more residential places of some kind, and it would be foolish to imagine that these can all be found outside the hospital service in the near future. At the same time that we expand community training and residential services, therefore, we must also be prepared to look more closely at existing hospitals and to give them the resources they need to develop better facilities, because they must carry the main burden of caring for the most severely retarded or handicapped patients.

7

CONCLUSIONS

Since the inauguration of the National Health Service in 1948, the number of subnormal patients in hospital has greatly increased. During the same period dissatisfaction has grown with the conditions under which most of these inpatients are cared for. Recently systematic examination of living conditions within subnormality hospitals, together with disclosures of malpractices in a few of them, have increased the pressure for reform.

One well conceived alternative to the present hospital system, the substitution of small residential units sited in urban areas, now receives official support. (D.H.S.S. 1971 a.) But the complete disappearance of the hospital is not envisaged and the proposed development programme is to be completed over a period of twenty years. In the meantime, many thousands of mentally handicapped people are living in grossly inadequate conditions and it is unthinkable that they should continue to endure such circumstances until an alternative system of residential care can be provided.

Sometimes improvements can be brought about through action taken in individual hospitals (Bavin, 1970). But if the majority of hospitalized patients are to benefit in the near future, action must be taken at regional or area level. This is not to argue that every Region, or Area Health Board, should adopt the same action. On the contrary, if different solutions are tried in different parts of the country, providing each is carefully monitored, it should be possible to assess the relative benefits and costs of each. But, whatever its form, for such action to be effective it must take account, as in the Wessex Region (Kushlick, 1967), of the particular characteristics of those patients who appear to require care in a residential setting. In other words any change must be based on knowledge of those handicaps and capacities of inpatients which are relevant to their medical, nursing training and occupational needs. Plans for reform, moreover, must be designed to allow for future modifications in the composition of this population, since there is no reason to suppose that this is stable.

The studies we have described were intended to contribute to this knowledge, which we believe to be necessary before reforms can be effective on a large scale. We have examined national statistics, described the characteristics of hospitalized patients in three Regions and sought to show how and why this population has changed within one area.

The first defect which became apparent was one of information. The review of published statistics on the hospital population, given in Chapter 2, shows that these were never very satisfactory. Until recently they have not covered the entire population of subnormals in hospital, and trends have often been confused by changes in the definition of the population. This was perhaps unavoidable, in some degree, for various administrative reasons, but there can be little justification for failing to state the nature of the changes or to comment on the irregularities in the trends. At the same time, too little information has been provided; the outstanding example is the absence of data on grade or handicap for inpatients or until recently on the extent to which patients are being trained or occupied. Equally, too little detail was provided about the characteristics of patients living in the community, or of those who were admitted to hospital, although the situation was improved with the publication of the Department of Health's Statistical Report series.

While we were working on these studies we came upon incidental evidence that the authorities responsible for local or regional administration of services kept their records in such a way that any information formally required by the (then) Ministry of Health was readily available, and that when figures were published relating to services in a particular area, it was usually the figures required by the Ministry which were used. In other words the returns required by the Ministry to a large extent determined what information was collected by the local administrators. Had the Ministry required more or different statistics as a routine, it is likely that records would have been arranged accordingly. It is important to realize that the information sought by central departments can also act as a useful guide at local level to the quality of care provided, especially if there is opportunity to make comparisons with other hospitals or areas. What seemed evident was that insufficient thought had been given at the centre to the use which could be made of national figures, and that few illuminating questions had been asked. Recent and considerable improvement has occurred, but it is still worth emphasizing that statistics collected regularly by government departments should be ones which are likely to provide information on the issues of major concern to the people professionally involved, which could also have an important educative function. For example, it would seem to be more important to have information which can be used to assess the burden on nursing resources or the adequacy of training facilities than information about the number of patients who are legally detained in hospital.

In the introductory chapter we stated some of the questions which seemed important in the context of determining present and future need. The first of these concerned the composition of the inpatient population and the relationship of grade and handicap to the availability of occupation and training. The study of hospital facilities reported in Chapter 3 indicated a low level of provision in educational and workshop facilities, and only very sketchy rehabilitation services. The more detailed examination of inpatients at ward level, described in Chapter 4, confirmed this conclusion. Perhaps as many as one-third of children who appeared to be eligible for it, in terms of their level of ability, were not in a school or receiving training, and at least 40 per cent of eligible adults were under-occupied or not occupied at all. We had no means of assessing the quality of the facilities for those in training, but other work suggests that the general standard of buildings and equipment is poor (Morris, 1969).

In this connection the transfer of the responsibility for the training of subnormals to the Department of Education and Science is to be welcomed. However, this policy perhaps carries the danger that, in the hospital setting, a rigid division could develop between the educational functions of the school, limited to one place and specific times, and the general functions of the ward, which ideally should be equally concerned with education. This is particularly important in view of our finding that some 28 per cent of medium- and high-grade children do not go to school, and, of course, very few indeed of the low-grade children do so.

If inpatients are to achieve their potential, two kinds of formal training programme should be provided, one type designed for those who are too low-grade or handicapped for anything other than sheltered workshop conditions, and another for those who with help might be able to work in the community. In order to achieve the latter objective, it is almost certainly necessary to work closely with the local community.

At the time this study was carried out, one of the main barriers to the provision of an effective service appeared to be the administrative division between local authority and hospital services. When we asked hospitals about liaison with their local Health and Education Departments, very little co-operation seemed to have occurred, and only a very few shared training facilities were mentioned. Our research was not designed to demonstrate this but we believe that more extensive co-operation or preferably integration of hospital and community services would improve facilities and also help to narrow the division between community and hospital care. (Owen *et al.*, 1968).

From 1974 the health service will be reorganized so that all health care will be unified under a single administrative system organized on a geographical basis under Area Health Boards. However, other administrative changes have now been introduced which will have the effect of splitting services for the mentally handicapped. The development of Area Health Boards could have made it possible to unite all forms of residential care, hospital and community homes and hostels, under a single administrative system, which would have facilitated flexible new developments in this field. However, from April 1971, the responsibility for the provision of local authority residential care was transferred from the Health Department to the Social Service Department, together with welfare and social work services, thus making close integration of hospital and community residential care more difficult to achieve. Another change is the transfer from the Health to the Education Department of responsibility for the education of mentally handicapped children. The provision of training and occupation for adults was transferred to the Social Service Department. While there are undisputed advantages in making schooling the responsibility of the Education Department, this division between departments for the education of adults and children could make an unfortunate break in the educational progression of the mentally handicapped.

It is obvious that to produce a good service for the mentally handicapped it is essential that the different departments integrate their efforts. Social Service Departments and Area Health Boards must work closely together both in the overall planning of residential care and in the decision to admit individuals or transfer them between the various forms of hospital, home or hostel care. Social workers in the community need to be consulted when residential care is being considered, particularly in the case of a discharge from hospital. It is also essential that training and education programmes for hospital residents and for those in the community be integrated, and that education services for children and adults be fully co-ordinated, especially since it would be entirely wrong if education were to cease at 16 or 18 merely for administrative reasons. We have argued in earlier chapters the need to educate the mentally handicapped beyond the conventional school leaving age.

If we are to learn anything from the experience of the past with the National Health Service, it is obvious that proper administrative machinery must be provided to effect liaison when three separately organized and financed services are involved. The establishment of collaborative machinery between the Area Health Boards, Social Service and Education Departments will not by itself ensure that a co-ordinated programme for the care and training of the mentally handicapped will be achieved. But experience with the health service seems to indicate that unless a system for collaboration is built into the structure it is unlikely to be realized. Only through such collaboration can we achieve the objective of retaining within the community all those mentally handicapped persons who are capable of leading a fairly independent life. A model scheme for integrating residential and training services is being undertaken in Sheffield, initiated by D.H.S.S., with the help of all existing authorities concerned. (D.H.S.S. 1971 b.) In some areas, particularly, close planning is needed immediately to ensure an even distribution of residential places between Areas, when the new local government and Area Health Board administrative divisions come into effect.

For many patients, however, rehabilitation into the community is not possible. We found that a minority of hospital residents, about 12 per cent, were very low-grade and that many of these patients were multiply handicapped. Furthermore, about a quarter of all inpatients had either a motor or a sensory handicap and about 55 per cent of all residents had been in hospital for over ten years. Even if these latter patients are quite high-grade, it is unrealistic to expect that many of them could be discharged to their own homes. For such patients, objectives must be more limited, but at the very least, they should be purposefully occupied during most of the day, and helped to become as independent as possible in attending to their basic needs.

We found in fact that about one-third of inpatients were unable to attend to one or more of their basic needs, but it seems likely that this proportion could be reduced if more attention were devoted to teaching patients to feed, dress and look after themselves, perhaps using Skinnerian techniques where necessary. This would, of course, be no simple task and would mean allocating more staff to the younger and more handicapped patients. It would also mean reorienting nurses towards training rather than care. But it would be rewarding work and in the long run it would release staff from feeding, dressing and cleaning older patients.

There is a very real challenge here. Nurses, like any other professional group, tend to see themselves in terms of the stereotyped images implied by their professional titles. The image of the nurse is of someone actively fighting to restore a sick person to health. When someone working in a subnormality hospital is called a nurse, he can scarcely fail to feel that his role is unglamorous and second-rate compared with that of the nurse in the acute wards of a general hospital. Nevertheless, he does see his role as a nursing one just because he carries the title, and in consequence he may not readily become involved in training activities within the ward. If new and more relevant roles are to be accepted, it will be necessary to reconstruct the self-image of the subnormality nurse, and this will involve a radical change in staff-training methods. Studies comparing the degree of institutionalization in different residential homes indicate that, where staff were child-care trained rather than nurse trained, the more anti-therapeutic features of residential life were avoided (King and Raynes, and Tizard, 1971). Where patients are treated on an individual basis rather than on a block basis, it is likely that they will more readily acquire the skills needed to achieve some independence.

There are some patients who may have the mental ability to care for themselves but who are perhaps unable to do so because of physical handicaps, and in these cases we suggest that mechanical aids should be evolved where possible and that much could be learned from the techniques developed for the physically disabled of normal intelligence. Again, the initial effort might be considerable in terms of staff time and equipment, but it would also mean that more staff would be involved in improving the patients' abilities and fewer in servicing them.

Our studies did not enable us to make any direct assessment of the quality of training and occupation provided for subnormal inpatients. However, the information we gathered on the age and grade of patients in hospital, on the prevalence of handicap, and on length of stay suggests the kind of questions which should be asked wherever facilities are being developed; for example, how many and which patients are likely to be in hospital or some form of residential care for most of their lives; what kind of training or occupation is appropriate for them and how should it differ from the training of those who will return to the community; or again, how many of the more handicapped patients could benefit from going to the school or training centre; and what kind of continuity could be developed between training on the ward and in the training centre. There is a need here for careful assessment at the individual level, and to plan or modify community as well as hospital services accordingly.

Hospitals could make a useful start by counting the number of patients unable to attend to themselves in various ways and assessing in some detail those who, with special training programmes, might be trained to look after themselves, and those who might do so if provided with mechanical aids. The task of assessment is ideally one for a team of specialists, but this would clearly be enormously costly in manpower alone. A great deal, however, could be done in a less ambitious way, if existing medical, nursing or psychological staff were to make assessments based on some simple questions, similar to the ones we asked. Assessments of this kind made on all the patients in a ward would provide a framework for training activities and allow staff to delineate reasonable targets for progress. Such an enterprise would clearly require the kind of co-operation and communication between staff of all kinds suggested by the Department of Health. (D.H.S.S. 1971 a).

It might indeed be found that nurses, however trained, are not the only people fitted for the task of teaching self-care and that they could well be supplemented by others, for example, unqualified but sympathetic housewives working part-time, under supervision: one hospital we visited did in fact successfully operate a scheme of this kind. In addition the various community service organizations to which many young people now devote some of their energies might also provide a useful source of ancillary help, as in some cases they have already done.

Some of the questions we asked in the introductory chapter concerned trends in hospital admissions and discharges, and the factors which influenced these trends. A study of admissions to the North-West Metropolitan Region described in Chapter 4 showed a marked increase in the number of patients entering hospital between 1949 and 1959, as did the national figures. Between 1959 and 1963, however, unlike the national figures, no further increase was apparent.

The whole period 1949–63 was marked by an accelerated rate of turnover in the Region, brought about by the expanded use of 'short-term' admissions, that is residential care specifically intended to last for under two months, and first introduced in 1952. This form of care was used particularly for younger patients. Comparing 1949 with two later years studied, there was actually a fall in long-term admissions, and the apparent increase in the numbers entering hospital occurred solely because of the extension of short-term care. While the total number of admissions increased therefore, the proportion of time patients spent in hospital, following first admission, decreased, due mainly to the large number of short-stay cases in the two later cohorts. In addition, patients admitted for long-term care also tended to spend rather less time in hospital in 1959 and 1963 than in the earlier year.

This suggests that, had we been able to extend the follow-up period beyond 1965, we would have found a decline in the number of patients actually resident. At a national level this decline occurred later, perhaps because community services in the country as a whole were not so advanced in development as in this area. However, there may be other factors making for increased admission rates for certain age groups, which will tend to diminish the decline in the hospital population, unless alternative services are introduced.

There were two groups of patients for whom long-term admission did not decline over the period studied. One consisted of low- and medium-grade patients over the age of 35 years, who had to be admitted, presumably, because elderly relatives were no longer able to cope with them at home. This type of admission is likely to increase further in the future, unless some form of hostel care is provided. The other group consisted of high-grade adolescents and adults. These patients were usually in hospital for a fairly short period and were discharged within six to nine months. However, 40 per cent of high-grade patients admitted in 1963 were still resident in hospital two years later, at the time of the follow-up. One would like to know more about these patients and why they were admitted to hospital in the first place, especially since an inadequate or broken home, or disturbed social behaviour, were reasons commonly given for long-term admissions in general. Do these patients need to be housed in hospital, and what characterizes those who cannot be discharged quickly? There is obviously a substantial demand for some form of residential care for inadequate or seriously disturbed adolescents and young adults, not necessarily permanently but certainly on a more than short-term basis. At present this need is being met by the subnormality hospital in the absence of any alternative, but if it is the aim of the psychiatric services to reduce the number of hospital patients, especially those who could be self-supporting, these are the most obvious candidates for placement in hostel accommodation. The possible functions of such hostels have been systematically explored in Lancashire (Campbell, 1968a and b), and these studies show that hostels can successfully deal with this type of patient.

To what extent was the overall decline in the volume of hospital care, which this study showed, due to improved community services? As far as the Region as a whole is concerned we cannot be certain. In Middlesex, however, where half the population of the Region lived, we were able to show that a decline in hospital admissions occurred simultaneously with the expansion of training-centre provision. This does not of itself, of course, prove that the expansion of training successfully diminished the pressure on hospitals. But since a decline in the *demand* for hospital care, that is including the numbers on the waiting-list as well as actual admissions, also occurred with the expansion of training facilities, this strongly suggests that the two trends did not merely coincide. Furthermore, looking at particular groups of patients we were able to show that, as services were increased for any one group, the demand for hospital services declined for that specific group. Of course even in a well-endowed area like Middlesex, the waiting-list for hospital admission did not dwindle to nothing, and in particular residential accommodation was still needed for children aged under fifteen. However, the experience of Middlesex is extremely encouraging in demonstrating the effectiveness of community services which are intelligently planned and generously provided. Research workers in the health and social services are all too familiar with well-intentioned experiments or innovations whose impact eludes any attempt at statistical validation. The success of the Middlesex experience is the more impressive since the subjective conviction of the innovators is borne out by the quantitative assessment of its results.

One important finding of our study is that there was no evidence of a difference in the characteristics of those children admitted for short-term care, i.e. specifically on a temporary basis, and those admitted for permanent care, and that half of the children admitted for short-term care were not on the waiting-list. This would seem to indicate that the grade or degree of handicap of the child is not the main factor in determining admission, and that when a high level of community service is provided together with generous arrangements for temporary care, many parents are willing to keep their severely subnormal children at home. The evidence is that at home children are likely to achieve a greater degree of independence than within the present hospital system (Tizard and Lyle, 1964). However, it seems unlikely that many of these children can be cared for at home indefinitely. Most of the low-grade and many of the medium-grade patients will eventually require the kind of care that few parents can willingly and easily give. From adolescence onwards it seems certain that increasing numbers of them will need residential placement of some kind. Even during the short period of our follow-up, a minority of patients first admitted on a purely temporary basis returned to the hospital later for permanent care. If this pattern is reflected nationally, then pressure for the admission of severely handicapped adolescents is likely to increase during the 1970s.

We feel very strongly that parents should be allowed a completely free choice as to whether or not they can accept the burden of bringing up their subnormal children. They should be told of the benefits to the child as well as the likelihood of the need, later, for hospitalization. Those who decide in favour of keeping their child at home should be supported in their resolve, emotionally and financially, as well as by the range of services of the type formerly provided by Middlesex. But if parents do not feel able to cope with such children at home, then some reasonable alternative should be provided, without blame or stigma being attached to their choice. It would be wrong to maintain these children in their homes against the real wishes of the parents and to the detriment of general family wellbeing. On the whole the evidence suggests that parents usually prefer to care for their children themselves, even at great emotional cost, but we must beware of a situation where they feel that they must do so for the benefit of the child, despite possible ill-effects to the other members of the family.

The best alternative for the care of children who cannot remain at home would seem to be small residential homes. However, if these are to be developed for the young it is important to consider what will happen to them when they arrive at adolescence. It will be hard to justify transferring these patients at the age of 16 to the existing hospitals with all their acknowledged deficiencies. Unless it is likely that in the near future all patients whose families cannot care for them will be housed for life in small residential units, it is important that the hospitals where they *will* be living are not neglected on the grounds that they do not provide the ideal form of residential care.

Some writers have argued as if it should be possible to

completely abolish hospitals for the mentally handicapped over the next ten or fifteen years and imply that to spend money on them now will only help to prolong their existence. (Franklin and Shearer, 1971). We believe this argument should be viewed with caution. While it might be unwise to base projections for the country as a whole on the experience of one area alone, it seems likely that the trends apparent in the North-West Metropolitan Region and in Middlesex are plausible indicators for future national trends. We have shown that it is certainly possible to reduce the demand for residential care when community services are improved, particularly for very young children, a group for whom community provision is still negligible in most areas. The services which seem to be most relevant are a flexible system of short-term residential care, combined with generous provision of pre-school and school-age care. For adults also the expansion of day care does seem to reduce the demand for residential placement.

But we have also shown that a large proportion of residents within hospitals have been there for so long or are so dependent that they are likely now to require closely supervised residential care for the rest of their lives. In addition, our results suggest that the number of hospital residents over the age of 55 years has increased greatly over the past 20 years and that the proportion of patients admitted aged over 35 years has also increased. Our cohort studies indicated a continued demand for residential care for high-grade adolescents, and we have predicted a possible future rise in the demand for residential care for medium and low-grade adolescents. The need for adult residential care is likely to remain considerable therefore. Much of this demand could be satisfied by community-based homes rather than hospitals, of course, but the number of places required makes it unlikely that these could be provided by the local authorities within the near future.

It is now generally accepted, as the White Paper implies, that very large or isolated hospitals simply do not make attractive homes for patients or for staff, and that even medium sized establishments should be broken up into small living units, particularly for children. Many of the existing hospital premises are far from ideal, some are totally unsuitable, and, of course, local authorities must be encouraged to provide alternative accommodation as quickly as possible. But meanwhile hospitals continue to carry the main burden of residential care, and it would be quite unfair to the present residents to stifle reform on the grounds that the institutions they inhabit may become obsolete at some unknown date in the future.

We have made few references to work carried out in other countries. On the research side there is, as far as we are aware, nothing which is directly comparable to the studies described here, although the inspiration for the cohort studies (Chapters 5 and 6) lies in the work of Kramer (1956, 1957, 1959) and Tarjan (1958) and their associates at the Pacific State Hospital, California. Those responsible for shaping the services of the future might well take into account the experience of other countries reviewed by Craft and Miles (1967). In particular, our interpretation of the findings of the inpatient survey (Chapter 4) implies a system of assessment and care similar to that developed in the U.S.S.R. for subnormals as described by Kety (1965). As Craft and Miles point out, the adoption of a similar system here would involve allocating considerably more resources to the care of the subnormal than at present. The argument that we should be prepared to do so was well made in the Report of the Committee of Inquiry into Allegations of Ill-Treatment . . . at Ely Hospital. The Committee suggested that the events at Ely were rooted in the poor physical and staffing conditions prevailing in the hospital, and that these are not necessarily peculiar to Ely alone.

Perhaps the essential point demonstrated by our enquiries is the great variation which exists between patients in their capacities and handicaps, and therefore in the kind of care they need. This is, of course, no new finding. It has been shown before by Leck and McKeown (1967), and by Kushlick (1968). It bears re-emphasis, because until the mentally handicapped population is recognized as differentiated, until each group within it and, ultimately, each individual is seen to require different treatment to enable him to live his life to the limits of his abilities, no substantial improvement can be expected.

It may be useful, finally, to consider the concept of patient 'needs' to which we have referred repeatedly, throughout this book. The needs we have specified are medical, nursing, training and occupational. This is neither an unusual nor an unreasonable selection, but it is to some extent arbitrary since there has been little study of what the mentally handicapped, especially the severely handicapped, do need. Needs must be related to ends, of course, and any system of care will inevitably have to serve many ends in addition to patient-oriented ones; the well-being of the patients' families, and of the wider community for example have also to be considered. But we feel that it is important, in devising any system of care, to specify each of these aims so that the means of achieving them can be reconciled one with another. Where ends conflict some compromise will be necessary, but the focus of the service must surely be the happiness or psychological well-being of the patient, and any development in the services must be assessed by this criterion primarily. For if this is not done and done continuously, it is difficult to see how the quality of the services can ever be systematically improved.

Although obviously a great deal of research effort remains to be undertaken before the optimum patterns of care can be achieved, there is now happily evidence that progress is not to wait on the optimal solution. The objectives are quite clear, and their achievement depends only on the diversion of sufficient resources. It is perhaps some measure of our relative sense of priorities that for the price of a few miles of urban motorway, all the improvements planned by the Department of Health could be implemented in the immediate future rather than over a period of twenty years.

APPENDIX 1

HOSPITAL COHORT - PROCEDURE

POPULATION COVERED

All first admissions to all National Health Service mental subnormality hospitals in the North-West Metropolitan Hospital Region for 1949, 1959 and 1963 were included. In addition, admissions to two non-N.H.S. hospitals with which the Regional Board has a contractual arrangement were included.

Admissions from the Region to one children's subnormality hospital outside the Region (Queen Mary's, Carshalton) were included in what proved to be the correct belief that a considerable number would have been admitted because the hospital was the only one of its kind in the south of England, and that these patients might differ from those admitted to hospitals within the Region.

Two hospitals in the Region which were not devoted exclusively to the care of the subnormal were included, because it was known that they regularly admitted subnormal children for short-term care.

Other hospitals in the Region which may occasionally take a patient for short-term care were not included.

Patients admitted from outside the Region were excluded unless they came from Central London. The latter were included on the assumption that a few patients on the borders of the Region in London might, at this time, have been admitted to hospitals in their own or the neighbouring Region.

Patients previously admitted to mental subnormality hospitals were excluded, and so also were patients previously admitted to psychiatric hospitals, except the Maudsley and Royal Bethlem hospitals. Previous admissions to psychiatric hospitals were excluded, because the behaviour which led to admissions there was believed to be similar to the behaviour which led to admission to a subnormality hospital. From the little information we had it seemed that the decision whether to admit, for example, a schizophrenic patient of low intelligence to a psychiatric or subnormality hospital was somewhat arbitrary.

Patients previously admitted to the Maudsley Hospital were included because it seemed that admission there was, for these patients, similar to an admission to a paediatric hospital, i.e. the purpose was mainly diagnostic and to provide intensive short-term treatment.

PROCEDURE

Names of all patients admitted either for long- or short-term care in the relevant years were extracted from hospital registers. All patients who had been transferred from another hospital or who had a record of a previous admission were excluded from the list. Later perusal of the hospital registers led to the removal of further patients as previous admissions. Since this perusal was for another purpose, we cannot be sure that no patient with a previous admission is included in the series, but the number should be very small.

A further visit was made to all hospitals in the series to record re-admissions of patients in the cohort to hospitals other than the one to which they were originally admitted.

Patients who were transferred from one of the hospitals concerned to a hospital outside the Region were thenceforth excluded from the cohort as 'left area'.

Our resources did not allow us to check the subsequent history of patients in the community, and for this reason there will be people whose loss from the original cohort is unrecorded (i.e. people who have died in the community or removed from the Region). This means that the depletion rates are likely to be inaccurate, particularly for the later cohorts, when a greater proportion of time was spent outside hospital. Evidence from the Local Health Authority cohort suggests that losses from deaths will be greatest year by year in the 1949 cohort, but nothing can be said about movement out of the Region, since Middlesex migration rates are not typical of the remainder of the Region (Census 1961).

Information extracted from case-notes covered :

Date of birth
Dates of all admission and discharges
Diagnosis
Grade, I.Q. when available
Other information on the patients' characteristics
Date of death or leaving area, if known
Source of admission
Reason for admission

Much of this information later proved to be unusable because details were recorded in such a small proportion of cases.

COHORT STUDY OF ADMISSIONS TO HOSPITAL

1.(a) *Year of cohort* 19...... 1(b) *Date of follow -up*..............

2. *Hospital*...

3. *Name of patient* ....

4. *Present status*—Not known   Y
                    In community care   X
                    In hospital   0
                    Discharged from care   1
                    Dead   2

5(a) *Patient's address at key admission*   (b) *Patient's last known address*
                                                  (if different from (a))
....
....
....

6. *Name of nearest relative* ....
    Relationship to patient ....
    Address (if different from 2(a) or 2(b))
(Fill this in only if   ....
patient has left   ....
hospital)   ....

7. *Father's occupation* ....

8. *Source of referral to hospital—*N.K. .... Y

   L.H.A X

   G.P. 0

   Police or Courts 1

   Other hospital or home
   (Specify) 2

   Other (Specify) 3

   ....

9. *Date of birth*

	ASCERTAINMENT			FIRST ADMISSION TO HOSPITAL			END OF CARE (*including follow-up*)		
	Date	Age	Time Interval	Date	Age	Time Interval	Date	Age	Time Interval
(a) Birth									
(b) First referral to L.H.A.									
(c) Ascertainment									
(d) First admission									

Reason for end of care....................................

10. *Diagnosis* ....
....
....
Physical handicaps ....
....
Behavioural disorders or emotional disturbances ....
....

11. I.Q. Test used Date

   ....

   ....

   ....

12. *Notes on previous history* (include information on schooling, employment and mental subnormality or illness in other members of patient's family)

13. *Hospital admissions*

	Date of admission	Date of discharge	Date of death	Length of stay
Key admission hospital	......	......	......	......
Previous admission hospital	......	......	......	......
	......	......	......	......
	......	......	......	......
Subsequent admission hospital	......	......	......	......
	......	......	......	......
	......	......	......	......
	......	......	......	......

Notes:
(a) Write T in red after date where discharge was a transfer out, and T in red, after date where admission was a transfer in.
(b) Write C in red before key admission and subsequent admissions which were compulsory.

14. *Admissions to other residential accommodation*

Type and address of accommodation	Date of admission	Date of discharge	Length of stay
Prior to key	......	......	......
	......	......	......
	......	......	......
	......	......	......
Subsequent to key	......	......	......
	......	......	......
	......	......	......
	......	......	......

15. *Date of death in community* ....

16. *Cause of death*...
....

(NOTE TO READER: In the actual Questionnaire a space for notes followed.)

APPENDIX 2

WARD QUESTIONNAIRE

POPULATION COVERED

Three hospital Regions were selected as stated in Chapter 4. Each subnormality hospital within the N.H.S. was included. The list of hospitals to be included was drawn up with the help of the Regional Boards, and on their advice we also included two private hospitals, in one Region, with a substantial number of contract beds.

We visited each hospital to be included in the study and drew up a one-in-ten sample using the ward registers as a base, rather than the inpatient register for the whole hospital, since this was likely to ensure a more representative sample by sex, age, and grade of patient. All patients resident in the hospital at the time of the survey (June 1965) were included even if they were temporarily absent from their wards.

PROCEDURE

As already stated, one of the authors visited each hospital in the study, and the nature and purpose of the survey was explained to the medical superintendent, the matron and the chief male nurse. The procedure for completing the questionnaire was explained to the nursing staff, who were asked to give the questionnaires for completion to the senior nurse on each ward. Notes for the guidance of nursing staff were printed on the questionnaire. On average each nurse would have to complete information on three patients, and rarely for more than five.

In a pilot study we tried to establish what questions to ask which would be meaningful to nurses, in addition to giving us the kind of material we required. In the main we limited ourselves to questions which the nurses could answer directly from their own experience and without having to consult case-notes, except of course for dates of birth and admission. Any question which seemed to cause problems at the pilot stage was explained more fully in the notes of guidance, and a brief account of the purpose of the questionnaire was printed on the outside cover, so that nurses would be informed about the nature of the survey and why we wanted this information. We indicated for which questions we thought it necessary to consult the ward doctor. A copy of the questionnaire follows.

The medical superintendent was asked to see that the completed forms were returned to us by post, and these were in almost every case returned very promptly. All the hospitals co-operated fully, and we are very grateful to all the staff concerned for their help.

WARD QUESTIONNAIRE

Region ....   Name of ward ....

Hospital ....   Total number of Patients
resident in Ward, June 1965.....

Purpose of the Questionnaire

This form is being sent out to every ward in all mental subnormality hospitals in three Regions, and from this we hope to build up a picture of the kinds of patients now in hospital in the whole country, which will be helpful in planning hospital staffing and accommodation in the future.

The form aims to give a very brief description of the patients' capacities and behaviour. It has been designed to collect this information with, we hope, the minimum of inconvenience to the ward staff. Because it has deliberately been kept brief, you may find difficulty occasionally in answering YES or NO to each question for a few patients. But it is very important that you do so and we have prepared some notes of guidance for questions which may pose some problems. These questions are marked with a star on the form.

THANK YOU VERY MUCH FOR YOUR HELP

Please answer YES or NO to each question below (except for Question 14).   Name of patient

Age or date of birth
Date of last admission
Sex (F or M)
*Estimate of grade

1. Patient is mongol.
2. Walks alone and unaided (if he needs help only on the stairs answer YES).

3. Can walk but only with help (if he is bedfast through sickness or old age, answer NO).
4. Normally feeds self, at least with a spoon.
*5. Is clean and dry both night and day (if he has occasional lapses, answer YES).
6. Is doubly incontinent, i.e. both of urine and faeces.
*7. Dresses himself, including buttons, alone and unaided
*8. Talks in sentences (of at least 3 words).
9. Tells time to within quarter of an hour.
10. Can read simple newspapers and magazines.
11. Can use both hands normally, i.e. has no paralysis, spasticity or uncontrolled movements of either hand.
*12. Patient is deaf (if he hears fairly well with a hearing aid and wears one answer NO).
*13. Patient is blind or nearly blind.
*14. How many epileptic fits has the patient had in the last 12 months (if none write O).
*15. Patient has a current prescription for anti-convulsants.
*16. Patient has current prescription for night sedation.
*17. Patient has a current prescription for day sedation or tranquillizers.
18. Is extremely overactive, e.g. paces up and down, does not sit still a minute.
19. Attacks others, e.g. hits out or bites, unprovoked or on very slight provocation.
*20. Constantly seeks attention. Is a great pest.
21. Is destructive, e.g. tears up newspapers and magazines, or destroys furniture.
22. Is continually injuring himself physically, e.g. head banging, picking at sores.
23. Patient is very withdrawn and solitary.
24. Goes to school each day for at least half the day.
25. Leaves hospital each day to work.
*26. Goes to work or O.T. on or off the ward at least 4 hours daily.
*27. Goes to work or O.T. on or off the ward at least 2 hours (but less than 4 hours) daily.
*28. Work or does O.T. sometimes.

WARD DOCTOR'S SIGNATURE ....

NURSE'S SIGNATURE.............. POSITION ON WARD..............

NOTE TO READER: In the actual Questionnaire columns were ruled vertically. The first for the Ward's reply and the second 'For Office Use'.

These questions should be answered by a ward sister or charge nurse who knows the patients well. The ward doctor should be consulted whenever this is possible on the estimate of grade and on questions 11 to 17.

We have prepared some Notes of Guidance which should clear up most of the difficulties which may arise in filling in the questionnaire. There is space below for you to write any comments that you wish about the questions or the patients.

(NOTE TO READER: In the actual Questionnaire a space for comments followed.)

NOTES OF GUIDANCE

Estimate of grade. This should be according to the old Mental Deficiency Acts (1913).

Write X for idiot (approx. I.Q. 0–25)

1 for imbecile (approx. I.Q. 25–50)

2 for feeble-minded (approx. I.Q. 50+)

5. 'Occasional' lapses, i.e. not more than once a week. Wetting or soiling which occurs during an epileptic fit should be regarded in the same way as ordinary wetting and soiling of any other kind.

7. 'Dresses alone'. If he needs help only with buckles and laces, answer YES.

8. If patient does talk a little, for example, odd words only, but can't string words together to make a sentence then answer NO to this question.

12. 'Patient is deaf'. By 'deaf' we mean cannot hear normal speech, i.e. is unable to respond to his own name because of deafness.

13. 'Nearly blind' means that, even with glasses, he cannot see to pick up smallish objects, about the size of a spoon.

14. Count only major fits, i.e. where the patient falls to the ground or loses full consciousness.

15, 16, 17. If the patient is receiving barbiturate as an anti-convulsant, answer YES to Question 15. In that case do not write YES for Questions 16 or 17, unless the patient is *also* receiving treatment as a sedative or tranquillizer.

18–23. If the patient's behaviour has changed recently, answer these items on his behaviour *over the last two months*, even if the change is due to drugs.

20. Every patient can be a nuisance at times, but here we mean those who are continually pestering for notice and attention.

24. A Junior Training Centre, or Special Care Unit, should be counted as 'a school'.

26, 27. 'Work or O.T.' includes industrial contract work, occupational therapy, hospital workshops, work on own or other wards, including helping with children's meals, etc.

'Daily' means at least 4 days a week.

28. 'Sometimes' means less than 2 hours a day, or less than 4 days a week. In other words, anyone who does some work or O.T. but cannot be included in 26 or 27.

THANK YOU VERY MUCH FOR YOUR HELP

APPENDIX 3

HOSPITAL SURVEY

Procedure

Regional Boards were asked to supply a list of all hospitals in their Region which were specialist hospitals for the mentally handicapped. The list did not include hospitals for the mentally ill or hospitals outside the N.H.S. with contract beds. The following Questionnaire was sent to each hospital named asking for some details of hospital residents and facilities.

HOSPITAL SURVEY QUESTIONNAIRE

REGION

HOSPITAL
(including the following units)

PART ONE

1. How many patients were resident in hospital at 31/12/64 (including patients on leave and temporary admissions)?

AGE	MALE	FEMALE	TOTAL
Under 16 years	......	......	......
16 years and over	......	......	......
Total	......	......	......

2. Can you give the number of these patients by grade – low, medium and high? If you cannot give a breakdown by sex and age, totals would be useful to us.

	LOW		MEDIUM		HIGH		TOTAL
I.Q. Approx	0–25		26–50		50+		
AGE	Male	Female	Male	Female	Male	Female	
Under 16 years	....	....	....	....	....	....	......
16 years and over	....	....	....	....	....	....	......
Total	....	....	....	....	....	....	......

N.B. We expect here an I.Q. estimate only. We realize that not all patients will have been tested, or at any rate not recently.

3. How many *direct* admissions were there to your hospital during the year ending 31/12/64? (Please do *not* include temporary admissions or transfers from other hospitals.)

4. How many temporary admissions (i.e. for short-term care as described in Ministry of Health Circular 5/52) were there during the year ending 31/12/64?

PART TWO

1. Do any of the patients in your hospital attend any of the following?

	In the hospital	Elsewhere
(a) Industrial contract work.	......	......
How many patients are involved?	......	......
(b) Occupational therapy, excluding (a).	......	......
How many patients are involved?	......	......
(c) A school or Junior Training Centre.	......	......
How many patients under 16 attend?	......	......
Do any patients 16 years and over attend and, if so, how many?	......	......
(d) Evening classes.	......	......
How many patients attend?	......	......
(e) Special care unit(s).	......	......
How many patients attend?	......	......

Please specify purpose. ....
....

2. Do any of your patients leave the hospital during the day to go out to work? If so, how many?

3. Do you have any nurses who are engaged primarily in training or educational activities rather than ward care, e.g. helping to run a workshop or O.T.? If so, how many and what work do they do?

4(a). Is there anyone in your hospital who is responsible for finding work for patients prior to or at discharge? If so, who?

4(b). Is anyone in the hospital responsible for finding accommodation for patients at discharge? If so, who?

5. Does your hospital have a social club for the patients and, if so, what kind of facilities does it provide, e.g. dancing, handiwork, etc.?

6. Does your hospital have a shop for patients within the hospital grounds?

7(a) Are any of your beds reserved exclusively for Temporary Admissions? If so, how many?

7(b) Are Temporary Admissions ever placed in other beds, e.g. of long-term patients on leave?

7(c). What do you see as the purpose(s) of temporary admissions? Please tick which item or items apply.

To provide accommodation for patients whilst parents take a holiday?
....

To provide accommodation for patients during a family emergency, e.g. mother's confinement? ....

To provide care for patients during a period of disturbed behaviour?
....

For assessment of patient? ....

Other (please specify) ....
....

8. Do you run an out-patient clinic? If so, for how many sessions a month?

What do you see as its purpose(s)? Please tick whichever item or items apply.

Diagnosis ....

Assessment...

Treatment...

Advice to parents on management ....

Reassurance and support for parents ....

Genetic counselling for parents ....

Other (please specify) ....
....

9. Is any building in your hospital used as a hostel? If so, what do you see as its main purposes? (If you have more than one hostel, please say how each is used.)

10. Is there any liaison or exchange of services between your hospital and the L.H.A. or L.E.A.? If so, please give details, e.g. do any of your patients attend training-centres or evening classes run by the local authority, or do patients living in the community share in hospital facilities?

11. Do you provide any services for your patients which have not already been mentioned?

12. What facilities, if any, which you do not already possess, would you like to see introduced into your hospital?

THANK YOU VERY MUCH FOR YOUR HELP

APPENDIX 4

L.H.A. COHORT – PROCEDURE

METHOD OF PROCEDURE

All patients referred as subnormal to the former Middlesex Local Health Authority during 1949, 1959 and 1963 were recorded.

These patients were selected from a punch card index system which enabled the names of all those patients referred in the relevant years to be extracted rapidly.

The indexing system was set up between 1952 and 1953, and some people who had died, left the area, been discharged or admitted to hospital during the two years following 1949 were omitted from the index system. These additional patients were found from a contemporary register.

A random sample of every second patient born less than sixteen years from the year of referral and of every fourth patient born sixteen years or more before was drawn from the lists compiled (which were arranged alphabetically).

The choice of a variable sampling fraction was made primarily on economic grounds : our resources did not permit us to study the entire cohort for each year nor to take a one in two sample of all patients. We chose a smaller sample of the older patients because we believed that there would be less variation amongst them in most of the variables with which we were concerned, and because our main interest lay in the experience of younger patients.

It would have been preferable to have had the dividing line between sampling fractions at precisely 16 years. But at the time the sample was drawn only the year of birth was known.

Numbers, as will be seen, were too small for each year to allow cross-tabulations of any complexity. An ideal design for the study might have taken all referrals in 1949–51, and compared them with those for 1959–61.

This sample yielded the following numbers: the actual numbers referred are given in brackets.

	1949	1959	1963
Under 16	97 (199)	107 (214)	107 (217)
16 and over	26 (108)	50 (209)	51 (203)
TOTAL	123 (307)	157 (423)	158 (420)

The case-notes for each patient were then used as sources for the following information :

Date of birth
Date of referral
Date when care ended (if before follow-up date)
Diagnosis – including information on ante- and perinatal events
Physical handicaps
I.Q. grade. Behavioural disorders or emotional disturbance
Dates of entering and leaving all forms of care within the
    follow-up period
Date of death, discharge or leaving area, if applicable

Not all case-notes included all the information; for example, information on ante- and perinatal factors was only available for a minority of cases. Dates were only absent in four cases (attendance at training-centres), but for these estimates could be made from other information.

If the case-notes showed that the patient had previously been referred to another Local Health Authority he was excluded from the cohort and not replaced.

This gave final numbers of patients as follows : weighted numbers are given in brackets.

	1949	1959	1963
Under 16	96 (192)	95 (190)	91 (182)
16 and over	22 (88)	42 (168)	43 (172)
TOTAL	118 (280)	137 (358)	134 (354)

For thirty-two patients in 1949, five in 1959 and three in 1963 no case-notes could be found and information had then to be extracted from the index cards. These should have provided full information on services received and d.o.b., but usually little diagnostic information, and no information on handicap and behavioural problems. For the eleven cases extracted from the register no information other than d.o.b., date of death or discharge, or admission to hospital was available. We assumed that none of these patients had received community services in the short time available.

When a patient was known to have been in contact with a general, paediatric or neurological hospital, additional information on diagnosis was obtained from the hospital concerned. In particular, this provided some information on four of the eleven patients drawn from the register. In addition, extra information was obtained for some patients, about whom little was known, from subnormality hospitals to which they had been admitted.

Information for each patient was entered on a schedule. Dates were translated into numbers of days since 1860 by means of a 'date and duration code' prepared by the Department of Epidemiology at Aberdeen University.

All other information was coded after rather than at extraction. This was partly because the quality of information available was not known until the study had begun, and partly because detailed enquiries were needed on the way in which medical information could best be coded.

Codings of both dates and characteristics were transferred to punch cards. Analysis of information was carried out on the University of London's Atlas computer. Calculations were programmed in Extended Mercury Autocode. Tabulations were derived through Multi-Variate Counter.

CLASSIFICATION OF PATIENTS' CHARACTERISTICS

1. Diagnosis

The final classifications made according to Heber (1961) were derived from a combination of definite diagnoses, information on structural anomalies, and factors of possible aetiological significance. The definite diagnoses considered were those where notes on records expressed no doubt that subnormality was due to

 (i) infection
 (ii) intoxication
 (iii) injury (at birth or later)
 (iv) disorder of metabolism
 (v) new growths
 (vi) mongolism
 (vii) other definite diagnosis, such as structural anomalies which included cranial anomalies, meningocele, and other cerebral defects (usually diagnosed at post mortem).

Factors of possible aetiological significance covered antenatal factors (e.g. maternal toxaemia of pregnancy, maternal rubella (where no definite diagnosis was made), birth factors (e.g. forceps delivery, mal presentation), multiple births, birth weight less than 5½lbs, head injury, infection, intoxication. The last three categories were used when there was no definite attribution of causality to the event by the doctor writing the casenotes, but where it was recorded that the patient's parents had claimed that the patient had deteriorated following the event).

For some patients more than one possible cause was recorded; in this case they were placed in the first category occurring in the classification.

2. *Physical disabilities*

(*a*) *Sensory impairment.* 'Blind' included those recorded as 'blind', 'partially or nearly blind' and '? Blind'. 'Deaf' similarly included 'deaf', 'partially deaf' and '? Deaf'.

(*b*) *Dependency.* Far more areas of ability were considered in making this rating – (i) ability to walk, (ii) continence, (iii) ability to feed self, at least with a spoon, (iv) ability to wash or dress self unaided.

Helpless patients were those stated to be so, or called 'cot cases' plus those who could not walk and were disabled in at least one other area, plus all patients of less than 18 months.

Almost helpless patients were those who could walk but had at least two other fields of disability recorded, plus those for whom it was only stated that they could not feed themselves, plus all patients of between 2½ and 5 years, unless there was evidence to the contrary.

At least some disability included all patients for whom only one area of disability (other than inability to feed self or walk) was stated.

Independent included all patients for whom this was stated, plus all feeble-minded patients over 5 years, and all mongols (who were not feeble-minded) over 10 years, unless there was evidence to the contrary, plus all patients who had been employed or attended an E.S.N. school.

(*c*) *Physical handicap.* These were patients who were handicapped by a deformity or disability which might make independence and particularly employment difficult even for a person of normal intelligence. The disabilities included were epilepsy, motor dysfunction, congenital abnormality, hydrocephalus, and blindness or deafness.

(*d*) *Congenital abnormalities.* The abnormalities included were:

   (i) congenital heart disease
  (ii) congenital cataract
 (iii) Spina bifida
 (iv) congenital dislocated hip
  (v) congenital kyphosis, scoliosis, kyphoscoliosis, torticulosis
 (vi) congenital talipes
(vii) other congenital abnormalities (e.g. cleft palate).

In practice it was not possible to be certain, in many cases, that the abnormalities mentioned were congenital. The assumption was always made that they were unless other evidence suggested that this was unwarranted. For example, kyphosis in an adult was not coded as a congenital abnormality.

Except for 'Dependency', coding of information extracted from case-notes on the dimensions described above was carried out by a recently qualified doctor.

COHORT STUDY OF PATIENTS ASCERTAINED

1(*a*)   *Year of cohort 19*......   1(*b*)   *Date of follow-up* ....

2.   *Name of patient*...

3. *Present status*—Not known   Y
                        In community care   X
                        In hospital   0
                        Discharged from care   1
                        Left area   2
                        Dead   3

4(*a*) *Patient's last known address*   4(*b*)   *G.L.C. borough No.* ......
       ....
       ....
       ....

5. *Name of nearest relative*.......................................
     Relationship to patient ....

6. *Father's occupation* ....

7. *Source of referral to L.H.A.*—N.K. ....Y
                        General or paediatric hospital.... X
                        Psychiatric or M.S.N. hospital......0
                        G.P. 1
                        L.E.A. 2
                        Police or Court 3
                        Other L.H.A. 4
                        Parents or guardian 5
                        Other (Specify) 6

DATE OF BIRTH	DATE OF ASCERTAINMENT
AGE	

Diagnosis ....
....
Physical handicaps ....
Behavioural disorders, or ....
Emotional disturbance..................................

I.Q.	Test used	Date
....	....	....
....	....	....
....	....	....
....	....	....

PT. NO. ....

SUMMARY SHEET

AGE at ascertainment
....

ASCERTAIN-MENT	HOSPITAL WAITING-LIST	TEMPORARY ADMISSIONS	LONG-TERM ADMISSIONS TO HOSPITAL	TRAINING-CENTRES	HOME TRAINING	HOSTEL ADMISSIONS	HOME VISITS	OTHER	END OF CARE

SUBSEQUENT HISTORY

1. *Hospital waiting list*

Date of entry	Date of leaving	Reason for leaving*
....	....	....
....	....	....
....	....	....

* Not known = Y,   Hospital admission = 1,   Death = 2,
Other service provided = 3,   Left area = 4,   Other = 5 (Specify).

2. *Temporary admissions*

Hospital	Date admitted	Date of leaving	Length of stay
....	....	....	....
....	....	....	....
....	....	....	....
....	....	....	....
....	....	....	....
....	....	....	....

3. *Long-term admission to hospital*

Hospital	Date admitted	Date of leaving	Length of stay
....	....	....	....
....	....	....	....
....	....	....	....
....	....	....	....
....	....	....	....

4. *Training centre attendance*

Training centre*	Date of entry	Date of leaving	Length of stay
....	....	....	....
....	....	....	....
....	....	....	....
....	....	....	....

* Not known = Y,   Junior = 1,   Adult = 2,   Mixed = 3,
Special care unit = 4,   Weekly boarding units = 5.

5. *Home training*

Days/week	Date of starting	Date of ending	Duration
....	....	....	....
....	....	....	....
....	....	....	....
....	....	....	....

6. *Hostel accommodation*

Hostel	Date admitted	Date of leaving	Length of stay
....	....	....	....
....	....	....	....
....	....	....	....

7. *Home visits*
Dates

8. *Reason for leaving care*

	Date	Reason
Discharged	....	....
Left area	....	....
Death	....	....
Whereabouts unknown	....	....
Other	....	....

BIBLIOGRAPHY

British Psychological Society, *Children in Hospitals for the Sub-normal: A Survey of Admissions and Educational Facilities* (London, 1966).

Brooke, E. M., 'A Census of Patients in Psychiatric Beds', 1963, Ministry of Health, *Reports on Medical Subjects* No. 116 (London, H.M.S.O., 1967).

Brown, G. W., Bone, M. R., Dalison, B. D. and Wing, J. K., *Schizophrenia and Social Care*, Maudsley Monograph No. 17 (London, 1966).

Brown, G. W. and Wing, J. K., 'A Comparative Clinical and Social Survey of Three Mental Hospitals', *Sociological Review*, Monogr. 5, Sociology and Medicine, eds P. Halmes and Keele.

Buchan, A. and Parry Jones, A., 'Cliffe View : A Six-Year Study of a Hostel for Subnormal Women', *Medical Officer*, Vol. 1 (1968), p. 41.

Bussey, A. and Wild, D., 'Mental Subnormality in West Sussex', *Medical Officer*, Vol. 1 (1969), p. 331.

Carter, C. O., 'A Life Table for Mongols with the Causes of Death', *Jour. Ment. Deficiency Res.*, Vol. 2 (1958), p. 64.

Castell, J. H. F., Clarke, A. D. B., Mittler, P. and Woodward, W. M., 'Report of the Working Party on Subnormality', *Bulletin of the British Psychological Society*, Vol. 16 (1963), No. 53, p. 37.

Campbell, A. C., 'The "Preventive" Use of Mental Health Hostels', *Medical Officer*, Vol. 120 (1968), p. 137.

— 'Characteristics of 352 Residents and 119 Ex-Residents of 14 Lancashire C.C. Hostels for Mentally Disordered Adults', *Medical Officer*, Vol. 1 (1968), p. 3.

— 'Family Contacts of Mentally Subnormal and Severely Subnormal Adults in Local Authority Hostels', *Medical Officer*, Vol. 122 (1969), p. 183.

— 'Comparison of Family and Community Contacts of Mentally Subnormal Adults in Hospital and in Local Authority Hostels', *Brit. J. Prev. Soc. Med.*, Vol. 22 (1968), p. 165.

Clarke, A. D. B., 'Genetic and Environmental Studies of Intelligence' in Clarke, A. D. B. and Clarke, A. M. (eds), *Mental Deficiency: A Changing Outlook* (London, Methuen, 1965).

Craft, M. and Miles, L., *Patterns of Care for the Mentally Subnormal* (Oxford, Pergamon Press, 1967).

Crome, L. in Hilliard, L. T. and Kirman, B. H., *Mental Deficiency*, 2nd ed. (London, Churchill, 1966).

Department of Health and Social Security, Annual Report, 1969.

Department of Health and Social Security, Statistical Report Series, 1969.

Department of Health and Social Security, Digest of Health Statistics, 1969.

Department of Health and Social Security, 'Better Services for the Mentally Handicapped'. H.M.S.O., 1971, Cmnd. 4683.

Department of Health and Social Security, 'Feasibility Study Report proposing a new pattern of service for mentally handicapped people in Sheffield County Borough'. 1971/MO (MS) 46/.

Farnklin, S. and Shearer, A., 'Future Services for the Mentally Handicapped' (Spastics Society, London, 1971).

Gordon, I., 'Seebohm Sophistry and Green Paper Gallimaufry', *The Lancet*, Vol. 1 (1969), p. 299.

Gruenberg, G. M., 'Epidemiology' in Stevens, H. A. and Heber, R. (eds), *Mental Retardation: A Review of Research* (University of Chicago Press, 1964).

Heber, R., *A Manual on Terminology and Classification in Mental Retardation*, 2nd ed., *Amer. J. Ment. Defic.*, Monogr. Supp. (1961), pp. 55–64.

Hilliard, L. T. and Kirman, B. H., *Mental Deficiency* (London, Churchill, 1965).

Jones, I., 'Community Accommodation for the Mentally Subnormal', *Brit. Hosp. J. and Social Service Review*, Vol. 2 (1967), p. 2,333.

King, R. D., Raynes, N. V., and Tizard, J., 'Patterns of Residential Care' (London, Routledge and Kegan Paul, 1971).

Kirman, B. H., 'Mentally Handicapped Persons', *British Medical Journal*, Vol. 2 (1968), p. 687.

Koch, R., Graliker, B., Bronston, W. and Fishler, K., 'Mental Retardation in Early Childhood', *Amer. J. Dis. Child.*, Vol. 109 (1965), p. 243.

Kaufman, M., 'The Effects of Institutionalization on Development of Stereotyped and Social Behaviours in Mental Defectives', *Amer. J. of Ment. Def.*, Vol. 71 (1967), No. 4, p. 581.

Krasner, L. and Ullman, L. (eds), *Research in Behaviour Modification* (Toronto, Holt, Rinehart and Winston, 1966).

Kushlick, A., 'A Method of Evaluating the Effectiveness of a

Community Health Service', *Soc. Econ. Admin.*, Vol. 1 (1967), No. 4.

— 'Care of the Mentally Subnormal', *The Lancet*, Vol. 2 (1969), p. 1,196.

Kushlick, A. and Cox, G. R., *Revision of Future Accommodation for the Mentally Subnormal*, Wessex Regional Hospital Board.

Leck, I., 'Changes in the Incidence of Neural Tube Defects', *The Lancet*, Vol. 2 (1966), p. 66.

Leck, I., Gordon, W. L. and McKeown, T., 'Medical and Social Needs of Patients in Hospitals for the Mentally Subnormal', *Brit. J. of Prev. and Soc. Medicine*, Vol. 21 (1967).

Leeson, J., *Demand for Care in Hospitals for the Mentally Subnormal* (a study conducted from the Department of Social and Preventive Medicine, University of Manchester, 1962).

— 'The Place of the Hospital in the Care of the Mentally Subnormal', *Brit. Med. J.*, Vol. 1 (1963), p. 713.

Lewis, E. O., 'Report of an Investigation into the Incidence of Mental Deficiency in Six Areas', 1925–7, Part 4 of *Report of the Mental Deficiency Committee* (H.M.S.O., 1929).

Lyle, J. G., 'The Effect of an Institution Environment Upon the Verbal Development of Institutional Children', Chapter 1 : Verbal Intelligence, *J. Ment. Defic. Res.*, Vol. 3 (1959), p. 122.

McCoull, G., A letter in *British Medical Journal*, Vol. 1 (1965), p. 191.

Mackay, H. and Sidman, M., *Instructing the Mentally Retarded in an Institutional Environment* (Proceedings of the Third International Symposium of the Kennedy Foundation, 1967).

Malamud, N., 'Neuropathology' in Stevens, H. A. and Heber, R., *Mental Retardation: A Review of Research* (University of Chicago Press, 1964).

Martin, F. M. and Rehin, G. F., *Towards Community Care* (London, P.E.P., 1969).

Mathers, J., 'Conditions in Psychiatric Hospitals', *The Lancet*, Vol. 1 (1969), p. 1,048.

Mawdsley, T., Rickham, P. P. and Roberts, J. R., 'Long Term Results of Early Operation on Open Myelomeningoceles and Encephaloceles', *British Medical Journal*, Vol. 1 (1967), p. 663.

Ministry of Health, Annual Reports, The Health and Welfare Services (1949–68).

— *A Hospital Plan for England and Wales* (London, H.M.S.O., 1962).

— *Health and Welfare – The Development of Community Care* (London, H.M.S.O., 1963).

— *National Health Service: The Administrative Structure of the Medical and Related Services in England and Wales*, the Green Paper (London, H.M.S.O., 1968).

— *Psychiatric Hospitals and Units in England and Wales* – In-patient Statistics from the Mental Health Enquiry for the Years 1964, 1965 and 1966 (Statistical Report Series No. 4, London, H.M.S.O., 1969).

Moncrieff, J., *Mental Subnormality in London: A Survey of Community Care* (London, P.E.P., 1966).

Morris, P., *Put Away: A Sociological Study of Institutions for the Mentally Retarded* (London, Routledge and Kegan Paul, 1969).

O'Connor, N. and Tizard, J., *The Social Problem of Mental Deficiency* (Oxford, Pergamon Press, 1954).

Owen, D., Spain, B. and Weever, N., *A Unified Health Service* (Oxford, Pergamon Press, 1968).

Pasamanick, B. and Lilienfeld, A. M., 'Association of Maternal and Foetal Factors with the Development of Mental Deficiency', I. Abnormalities in the Pre-natal and Paranatal Periods, *Journal American Medical Association*, Vol. 15 (1955).

Pilkington, T. I., 'Hospital Services for the Subnormal', *The Lancet*, Vol. 2 (1963), p. 992.

Primrose, D. A. A., 'Natural History of Mental Deficiency in a Hospital Group and in the Community It Serves', *Journal of Mental Deficiency Research*, Vol. 10 (1966), Part 3, p. 159.

Registrar General's Statistical Review of England and Wales, Supplement on Mental Health, 1949–1960 (London, H.M.S.O.).

Rehin, G. F., 'Community Mental Health Services and the See-bohm Report, *Medical Officer*, Vol. 1 (1969), p. 135.

Rehin, G. F. and Martin, F. M., *Psychiatric Services in 1975* (London, P.E.P., 1963).

Report of the Committee of Inquiry into Allegation of Ill-Treatment of Patients and Other Irregularities at the Ely Hospital, Cardiff, The Ely Report (London, H.M.S.O., Cmnd 3975, 1969).

Royal Commission on the Law Relating to Mental Illness and Mental Deficiency, 1954, 1955, *Minutes of Evidence* (London,

— *Report* on the Law Relating to Mental Illness and Mental Deficiency, 1957 (London, H.M.S.O.).

Sabagh, G. and Windle, C., 'Recent Trends in Institutionalization Rates of Mental Defectives in the United States', *American*

Journal of Mental Deficiency, Vol. 64 (1959), No. 4, pp. 618–23.

Shapiro, A., 'Hospital Services for the Subnormal' (A letter), *The Lancet*, Vol. 2 (1963), p. 1,165.

— 'Care of the Mentally Subnormal', *The Lancet*, Vol. 2 (1969), p. 957.

Sidman, M. and Stoddard, L. T., 'Progamming Perception and Learning for Retarded Children', in Ellis, N. R. (ed), *International Review of Research in Mental Retardation* (New York, Academic Press, 1966).

Stein, Z. and Susser, M., 'Estimating Hostel Needs for Backward Citizens', *The Lancet*, Vol. 2 (1960), p. 486.

— 'The Families of Dull Children : A Classification for Predicting Cancers', *British Journal of Prev. and Soc. Medicine*, Vol. 14 (1960), No. 2, p. 83.

Stephens, E. and Robertson, J., 'Growing Up in Hospital'. In 'Mental Retardation Occasional Papers' (London, Butterworth, 1972. In press). Published for the National Institute for Research into Mental Retardation.

Tarjan, G., Dingman, H. and Miller, C., 'Statistical Expectations of Selected Handicaps in the Mentally Retarded', *Amer. Jour. Ment. Def.*, Vol. 65 (1960), No. 3, p. 335.

Tizard, J., *Community Services for the Mentally Handicapped* (London, Oxford University Press, 1964).

— Introduction in Clarke, A. and Clarke, A. D. B. (eds), *Mental Deficiency: A Changing Outlook*, 2nd ed. (London, Methuen, 1965).

Tizard, J. and Grad, J. C., *The Mentally Handicapped and Their Families: A Social Survey* (London, Oxford University Press, 1961).

Tizard, J., King, R. D., Raynes, N. V. and Yule, W., *What is Special Education?* Proc. Int. Cent. Ass. Special Education (London, 1966), pp. 24–8.

Tarjan, G., Dingman, H. and Miller, C., 'Statistical Expectation of Selected Handicaps in the Mentally Retarded', *Amer. Jour. Ment. Def.*, Vol. 65 (1960), No. 3, p. 335.

Ullman, L. and Krasner, L., *Case Studies in Behaviour Modification* (New York, Holt, Rinehart and Winston, 1965).

INDEX

Printed and bound by CPI Group (UK) Ltd, Croydon, CR0 4YY

23/10/2024

01777998-0001